APPLIED
CORE CONDITIONING

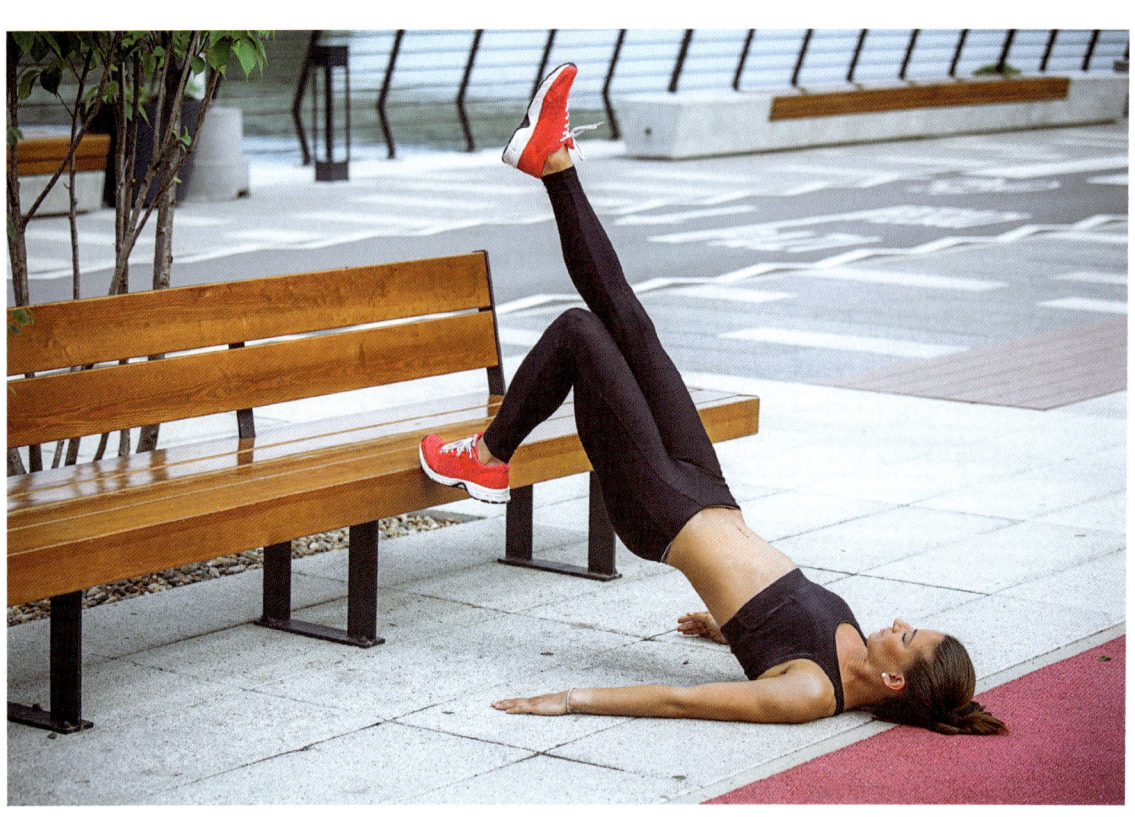

APPLIED
CORE CONDITIONING

ALEX REID

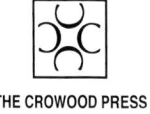

THE CROWOOD PRESS

First published in 2018 by
The Crowood Press Ltd
Ramsbury, Marlborough
Wiltshire SN8 2HR

www.crowood.com

© Alex Reid 2018

All rights reserved. No part of this publication may be reproduced or transmitted in any form or by any means, electronic or mechanical, including photocopy, recording, or any information storage and retrieval system, without permission in writing from the publishers.

British Library Cataloguing-in-Publication Data
A catalogue record for this book is available from the British Library.

ISBN 978 1 78500 521 3

Dedication
For Malc. For Mum. For Dad. Thank you.

Typeset by Servis Filmsetting Ltd, Stockport, Cheshire

Printed and bound in India by Parksons Graphics

CONTENTS

Acknowledgements		6
Getting Through This		7
1	Introduction: What is the Core? Why is it Important?	8
2	Musculoskeletal Disorders: The Financial Cost and Possible Solutions	34
3	Case Studies: The Practical Application of Core Conditioning, Prescription and Exercise Selection	43
4	Applied Core Conditioning: Programming, Prescription and Sports-Specific Training	111
5	Summary	165
Glossary		169
References		171
Index		174

ACKNOWLEDGEMENTS

Thank you to the following contributors within this book. Your efforts and the time given to help bring things together are greatly appreciated:

Core, anatomy and muscular images: Visualcoaching Pro (visualcoaching.com); Photography: Peter Court Media Services

The case studies in this book are anonymous, but I would like to thank my clients, who have provided me with insight and experience, and inspired me to provide optimal conditioning, rehabilitation and reconditioning programmes for them.

I would also like to thank my family, particularly Isla and Machrie, as well as my friends who have encouraged and supported me during the writing and creation of this book.

GETTING THROUGH THIS

I was asked to write this foreword as a fairly average person who was fit and healthy and worked hard at a lot of different things. I started running in my early thirties and quickly challenged myself to get faster and faster. I pushed myself quite hard and was fairly happy with my personal bests at 10k and half-marathon distances. Then, when I was thirty-five I ruptured my anterior cruciate ligament playing a bounce game of 5-a-side football. I went home after the game thinking I had done something bad. It was diagnosed by the physio the next day and all was confirmed by a MRI scan a couple of days later. I had little knowledge of the severity of this injury until I started my rehabilitation. Notwithstanding a second operation due to receiving an infection during my first operation, the journey back to running was an arduous, year-long, pain-threshold-extending challenge. I've never recovered fully from this and, with the exception of a burst of activity to beat my 10k personal best, I've never got near my old cadence.

In 2017, six years after my ACL repair, I suffered a prolapsed disc in my lower back. Anyone who has ever experienced this (and you may well have if you're taking the time to read this book) will know the pain a body can go through. The ACL injury was nothing in comparison. Prolapsed discs don't usually happen because of a one-off episode. Instead, they usually build up over a prolonged period of time. I put mine down to a few years of imbalance after losing the ability to bend my right knee properly following the two ACL operations. Not being strong enough in my lower back, having poor posture and indulging in some rather savage sessions removing bamboo from our front drive, all conspired to create the perfect storm.

Six months after the prolapsed disc diagnosis, I am now able to run again, but those six months have been torture. It affects everything. Even trying to move an inch in bed is difficult. Your head thinks about your posture the whole day. It gets to you. You can't sit with your family and have a bit of fun. You can't lie on the floor, sit on a chair, cross the road fast, sit at your PC. You walk along the road and spasm. You stare at seats on the train trying to work out how to sit on them.

The only way you can recover is by getting stronger and preventing it from happening again. The core is the key. Every exercise that strengthens your trunk brings you one step closer to shaking off vulnerability. From my ACL recovery and strengthening everything around the knee, my focus has now shifted to strengthening my core. If only this book had already been written, and I had started earlier!

Anonymous

CHAPTER 1

INTRODUCTION: WHAT IS THE CORE? WHY IS IT IMPORTANT?

As you sit reading this, you will be subconsciously activating your abdominal muscles and trunk, commonly referred to as your 'core'. Without this activation, our skeleton would be floppy, our spine unsupported and our overall function compromised. The muscles around our mid-section or trunk are constantly working to allow locomotion, smooth movement, control and function, and the activities that we do constantly demand this activation from the muscles involved.

Beth West, one of my good friends, posted the following on social media whilst on her journey to work in London one day in 2017:

> *Commuting on Southwest Trains of a morning is a tough core workout. Too crowded to be able to reach anything to hold on to, you must use your core to ensure that you are not toppling on to fellow passengers. They should market that. Maybe put some personal trainers on carriages and make it a proper workout!*

A true reflection of the day-to-day challenges placed upon us all, it made me laugh out loud. Our core, lumbar spine, glutes, pelvis and associated limbs are constantly in use during our working day, with numerous actions requiring strength and control. When standing on a busy commuter train, we must stabilize and control our body all the time, in order not to fall on to the person next to us. It is a good example of a chaotic environment that we need to control, just like sport or lifting or working in a physical job. Every day, we place many demands on our body and expect it to cope. Sometimes we forget that, although the human body is made to work and move, if it is not properly conditioned, then injury is likely.

The body works as a global, combined unit. Despite a limb moving, it may appear, independently, on the contrary the movement is as a result of a number of combined, coordinated actions within the body: a neural, muscular, metabolic, conscious and subconscious decision to complete a movement made by a reaction to a stimulus, by choice, or sometimes involuntary, like reacting to a sudden move on that busy train, or reaching instinctively to catch something as it falls, or playing catch with your kids. It is very complex, but it works seamlessly on most occasions and allows us to be the mobile, skilled, dexterous beings that we are.

But what happens if we get injured? What if we are not strong enough to cope with these demands or have bad posture, which leads to pain and immobility? What if there is a leg-length discrepancy, which may lead to poor biomechanics and resultant back pain, or an over-use injury as a result of a muscular imbalance? How in those cases do we address the day-to-day issues and challenges? The solution lies in becoming stronger and better

INTRODUCTION: WHAT IS THE CORE? WHY IS IT IMPORTANT?

conditioned, ensuring good mobility, retraining our movement patterns, and reintroducing effective and efficient activation of the trunk and core musculature.

The muscles around the abdominal region, known widely as the core musculature, originate and insert within the axial skeletal system and link through to the appendicular skeleton. They are the link in the chain that coordinates our movement. Without them, movement would be clumsy and uncoordinated. The body works well as a unit, but sometimes it needs to be retrained and re-educated to take care of itself. It is very easy for it to become lazy, to adopt bad habits and become deactivated, which can cause problems. Often the larger, more dominant muscles are recruited before the more appropriate, synergistic muscles. This poor muscle recruitment can lead to an imbalance and over-use.

The lifestyle choices that many people make in this time of high technology – sitting for hours playing games, using social media or messaging on their devices – can cause a deconditioning of the body and, potentially, long-term health issues. Prolonged use of and addiction to mobile phones and hand-held devices lead to poor posture and bad habits, which can cause muscular over-use and pain.

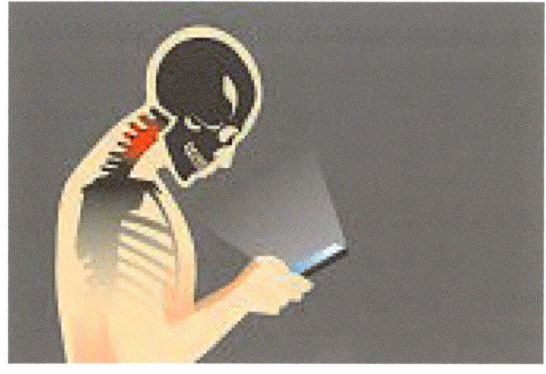

Prolonged use of smart phones and hand-held devices often lead to poor posture and resultant neck pain.

Similarly, drivers who commute to work by car, or drive for a living, can also suffer health problems, as a result of sitting in a flexed position for many hours, often with poor posture and with the neck tilted forward. We have all got out a car after a long journey and felt stiff and sore because of the position we have been in for the past few hours. The effect is exacerbated for those who drive day after day, for lengthy periods. They can experience all sorts of issues, including a reduction in muscle length and postural imbalances, as well as weight gain, which can of course lead to other health issues, such as obesity, high blood pressure and diabetes.

The body likes to work. It is happier being active and also healthier. Detraining often causes problems in a body that craves action. Inactivity and poor posture and biomechanics can cause long-term problems, which lead to pain and immobility. However, good posture and positioning, and a core and trunk that activate well on demand and in sequence, allow the body to move effectively and without pain. If an individual's capacity to control the body's movements is compromised by injury, illness, detraining, bad habits, bad posture or extreme overload, things may well start to break down and cause pain.

There is a high incidence of low back pain in a number of groups, including the obese, low-income, elderly and middle-aged populations, as well as those in occupations such as firefighting, baggage-handling, health care, long-haul and taxi driving and office work, who are sitting for prolonged periods of time, or lifting and rotating, pushing and pulling as part of their daily activities. Chronic pain may lead to further problems, such as depression and mental health issues, as well as the inability to work, which affects not only the individual in pain, but the whole family. It is a massive worldwide problem.

The link between pain and depression and depression and pain has been the subject of much research. In a 2004 paper, Madhukar H. Trivedi, MD, discussed the incidence of pain and depression

INTRODUCTION: WHAT IS THE CORE? WHY IS IT IMPORTANT?

and the similarities. Major depression is also associated with painful physical symptoms such as headache, backache, stomach ache, joint ache and muscle ache. Because depression and pain share a common neuro-chemical pathway, in that they are both influenced by serotonin and norepinephrine, depression and associated painful physical symptoms must be treated together in order to achieve remission (Madhukar H. Trivedi, M.D, 2004).

Depression can present itself as pain in the body and it also seems to be the case that chronic pain can lead to depression or mental health issues, creating a vicious cycle. Research by Denniger *et al.* (2002) has also shown that physical symptom improvement was correlated with the improvement of other depression symptoms. This suggests that the patient's ability to achieve depression remission may be directly related to the reduction of painful physical symptoms. Therefore, it appears to be a cyclical problem:

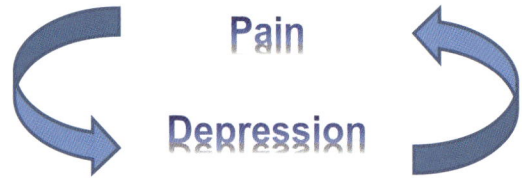

If pain can be reduced, mental health issues can hopefully be affected in a positive way. The challenge is the worry that any remission may be temporary and that the problem may come back with another painful debilitating onset. This is where an effective and efficient conditioning programme can help, in removing any concerns about future pain, inhibition or loss of function.

The trunk and the core protect and stabilize the axial skeleton, to allow it to function free from pain; if this is compromised at all, problems may occur. The aim of this book is to provide a useful resource that will help you to become more applied in the prescription and programming of appropriate core-conditioning strategies, to allow you to stay fit and have a healthy spine, prevent injury by ensuring appropriate conditioning of the core. It should be suitable for performance athletes, sedentary populations, as well as those who have had the unfortunate experience of low back pain and associated injury.

There are many other resources available, with exercises and guidelines to follow, but the approach here is slightly different, in that it is more applied. Chapter 3 presents a number of case studies, relating to some of the most common injuries, including prolapsed disc, pars defect, groin strain, piriformis syndrome, hamstring tendinopathy and diastasis recti. In each case study, an applied conditioning plan has been devised, based upon real challenges and issues, and this can be used to identify appropriate exercises to address common and often debilitating problems in an applied setting.

The case studies, along with the sports-specific conditioning explained in Chapter 4, will help with exercise selection, prescription and programme design. The sports-specific exercises in Chapter 4 will help ensure a strong, robust core, which should reduce the potential for injury and enhance performance. They cover the whole range, from foundation, isometric exercises to more functional, whole-body demands. Sets, repetitions and loading are all discussed in detail.

THE SKELETAL AND MUSCULAR SYSTEM

The skeletal system in an adult body is made up of 206 individual bones. These bones are arranged into two major areas within the skeletal system: the axial skeleton and the appendicular skeleton.

The axial skeleton (the bones of the head and trunk) runs along the body's midline axis and is made up of 80 bones in the following regions:

- Skull
- Hyoid
- Auditory ossicles

INTRODUCTION: WHAT IS THE CORE? WHY IS IT IMPORTANT?

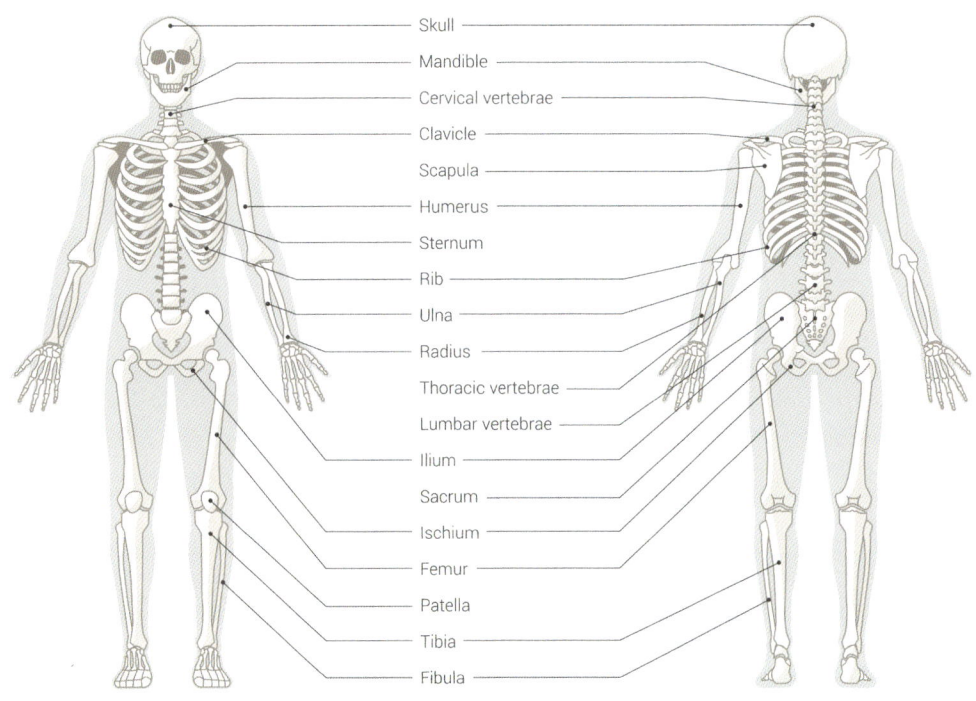

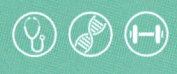

The Skeletal System
Human Body Systems

Skeletal system.

- Ribs
- Sternum
- Vertebral column

The appendicular skeleton is made up of 126 bones in the following regions:

- Upper limbs
- Lower limbs
- Pelvic girdle
- Pectoral (shoulder) girdle

The axial skeleton and the appendicular skeleton are connected via connective tissue, such as fascia, ligaments, tendons and muscles, making up the global unit within the body that allows coordinated movement. For reference within this book, the core and trunk musculature includes both the axial skeleton, specifically the vertebral column, and the appendicular skeleton, specifically the pelvic girdle and lower limbs. These work in unison to allow functional and specific movement patterns for effective locomotion and stability.

The bony framework of 206 bones – 80 axial or trunk bones and 126 bones of the limbs (appendicular) – does not include teeth or sesamoid bones other than the patella. The location of these bones is presented below.

INTRODUCTION: WHAT IS THE CORE? WHY IS IT IMPORTANT?

Axial (80 bones)		Appendicular (126 bones)	
Head	**Trunk**	**Upper extremities**	**Lower extremities**
(29 bones)	(51 bones)	(64 bones)	(62 bones)
Cranial 8 Frontal 1 Parietal 2 Occipital 1 Temporal 2 Sphenoid 1 Ethmoid 1 *Facial 14* Maxilla 2 Mandible 1 Zygoma 2 Lacrimal 2 Nasal 2 Turbinate 2 Vomer 1 Palatine 2 *Hyoid 1 Auditory ossicles 6* Malleus 2 Incus 2 Stapes 2	*Vertebrae 26* Cervical 7 Thoracic 12 Lumbar 5 Sacrum 1 Coccyx 1 *Ribs 24* True rib 14 False rib 6 Floating rib 4 *Sternum 1*	*Arms and shoulders 10* Clavicle 2 Scapula 2 Humerus 2 Radius 2 Ulna 2 *Wrists 16* Scaphoid 2 Lunate 2 Triquetrum 2 Pisiform 2 Trapezium 2 Trapezoid 2 Capitate 2 Hamate 2 *Hands 38* Metacarpal 10 Phalanx (finger bones) 28	*Legs and hips 10* Innominate or hip bone (fusion of the ilium, ischium, and pubis) 2 Femur 2 Tibia 2 Fibula 2 Patella (kneecap) 2 *Ankles 14* Talus 2 Calcaneus (heel bone) 2 Navicular 2 Cuboid 2 Cuneiform, internal 2 Cuneiform, middle 2 Cuneiform, external 2 *Feet 38* Metatarsal 10 Phalanx (toe bones) 28

(http://medical-dictionary.thefreedictionary.com/axial+skeleton)

As the case studies and sport-specific exercises will show, many muscles in the lower limbs cross over between the appendicular and axial skeleton and are therefore vital in establishing a stable, strong body and core. The exercises within the conditioning programmes have been selected often both for core function and for their overall benefit to functional movement and performance. Many whole-body exercises are also included, which challenge the core and create a more functional outcome.

Movement within the skeletal system is achieved by the use of levers. In the human body, the joints act as a fulcrum and the bones as the levers. As one muscle shortens, the opposite muscle will lengthen with concentric or eccentric movement. This is the basic concept of a lever within the human body, using agonist and antagonist muscles.

There are three types of lever used within the human body: first class, second class and third class. They are defined by the relative position of three elements of the lever: the effort (E), the position of the fulcrum (F) and the load or resistance (R).

The muscles attach to the skeleton via tendons and as a muscle shortens through a contraction it will cause movement along the lever or a contraction of the muscle. It is necessary to have a fulcrum to work with the lever to allow for movement. The core musculature, around the spine and vertebral column and pelvic girdle, generally works as a stabilizer without an obvious single lever in place. Unlike a biceps curl, for example, which involves an agonist and antagonist muscle action during the flexion of the arm, the core musculature acts to stabilize in a constant manner, based upon its muscle fibre type, to allow multi-directional, controlled movement. It is like a cylinder that allows free-flowing rotation, flexion, lateral flexion and extension around the pelvic girdle, lower limbs and vertebral column. This concept of a cylinder around the spine explains why this area of the body is known as 'the core'.

In order to plan and programme different exercises, it is important to recognize the different types of muscles and tissues around the core and to consider their function. Based upon certain structural and functional characteristics, muscle tissue is classified into three types: cardiac, smooth and skeletal.

- Skeletal muscle (or striated muscle) is responsible for locomotion and general movement. Skeletal muscle tissue can be made to contract or relax by conscious control so its engagement is generally voluntary.
- Cardiac muscle (relating to the heart): contraction of this type is completed without thinking about the muscular action and is therefore involuntary.

INTRODUCTION: WHAT IS THE CORE? WHY IS IT IMPORTANT?

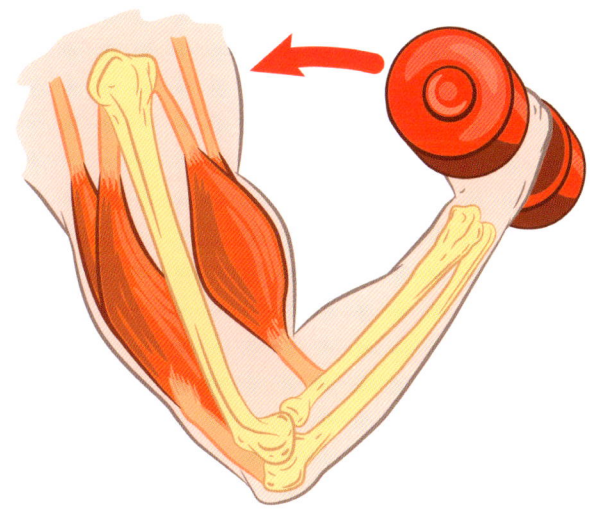

Example of a lever: biceps curl.

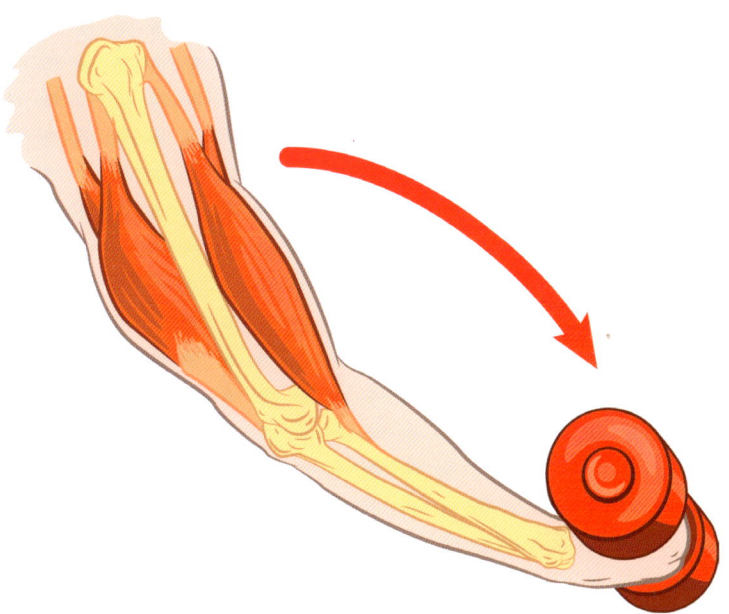

- Smooth muscle (also an involuntary muscle) lines the walls of the arteries to control blood pressure, and controls the digestion of food by causing movement of the intestine and the urinary bladder, for example.

Fascia is the soft-tissue component of the connective tissue system and is another important structure within the skeletal system, particularly around the core musculature. It interpenetrates and surrounds muscles, bones, organs, nerves, blood vessels and other structures. It is an uninterrupted, three-dimensional web of tissue that extends from head to toe, from front to back, from interior to exterior (Fascia Research Congress, 2009).

Fascia is responsible for maintaining the structural integrity of the skeleton and for providing support and protection. It also acts as a shock absorber.

INTRODUCTION: WHAT IS THE CORE? WHY IS IT IMPORTANT?

Types of Muscle

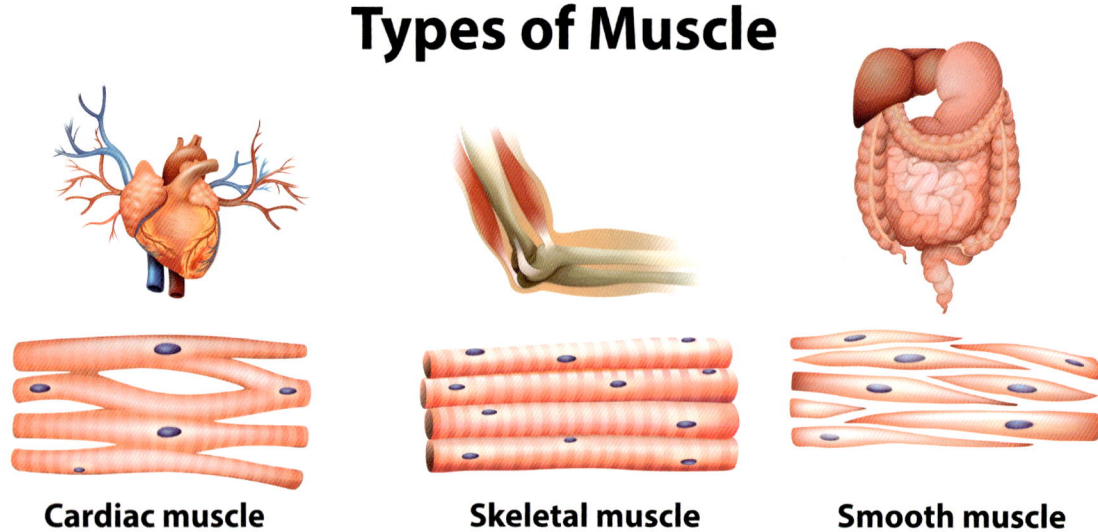

Types of muscle: cardiac, skeletal and smooth muscle.

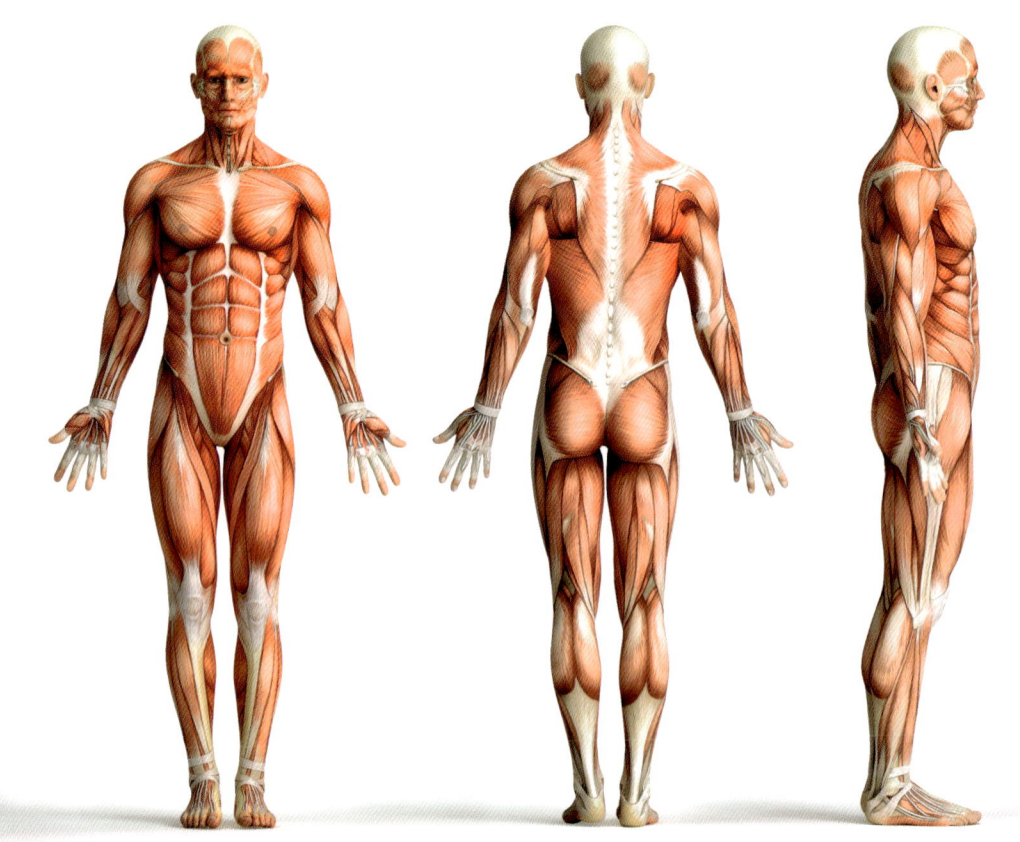

Fascia: the depicted white areas are fascia within the skeletal system.

INTRODUCTION: WHAT IS THE CORE? WHY IS IT IMPORTANT?

There is a significant amount of fascia around the core area within the axial and appendicular skeleton.

Skeletal muscles contain thousands of muscle cells, or muscle fibres, which run from one tendon to the other. They have a capacity to contract and extend, which allows for movement. There are three main types of muscle fibre – Type I, Type IIA and Type IIB – and each one has a specific role within muscular function.

Muscles of the shoulders and arms are not constantly active but are used intermittently, usually for short periods, to produce large amounts of tension, as in lifting and throwing. These muscles have a higher proportion of Type I and Type IIB fibres. Most skeletal muscles within the body however are a mixture of all three types of fibre, with the proportion varying according to the action of the muscle. For example, the postural muscles of the neck, back and legs have a higher proportion of Type I fibres, which means they are aerobic in nature and have a high resistance to fatigue. This allows them to function at a constant activity level; they are often referred to as tonic muscles.

The core musculature is dominant in this category of muscles that have a high proportion of slow-contracting Type I fibres. It is capable of remaining tonic to support the spine and lumbo-pelvic region as the body moves, and has a high resistance to fatigue with a low force production. It is only when an increased demand is placed upon the region that the Type IIA and Type IIB fibres kick in, to increase strength and activation. As the Type IIA and IIB fibres have a lower resistance to fatigue, when those muscles are called into action with specific core exercises, the body will feel the effect – like the 'burn' experienced after completing a large number of sit-ups!

Even though most skeletal muscle has a mixture of all three types of muscle fibre, all the skeletal muscle fibres of any one motor unit are all the same. In addition, the different skeletal muscle fibres in a muscle may be used in different ways, depending on the requirement or demands placed upon it. For example, if a task demands only a weak contraction, only Type I fibres will be activated by their motor units. If a stronger contraction is needed, the motor units of Type IIA fibres will be activated. If a maximal contraction is required, motor units of Type IIB fibres will be activated as well. It depends on supply and demand. Activation of various motor units is determined in the brain and in the spinal cord. Although the number of the different skeletal muscle fibres does not change, the

Fibre Type:	Type I fibres	Type IIA fibres	Type IIB fibres
Contraction time	Slow	Fast	Very fast
Size of motor neuron	Small	Large	Very large
Resistance to fatigue	High	Intermediate	Low
Activity Used for	Aerobic	Long-term anaerobic	Short-term anaerobic
Force production	Low	High	Very high
Mitochondrial density	High	High	Low
Capillary density	High	Intermediate	Low
Oxidative capacity	High	High	Low
Glycolytic capacity	Low	High	High
Major storage fuel	Triglycerides	CP, Glycogen	CP, Glycogen

(BrianMac Sports Coach: http://www.brianmac.co.uk)

INTRODUCTION: WHAT IS THE CORE? WHY IS IT IMPORTANT?

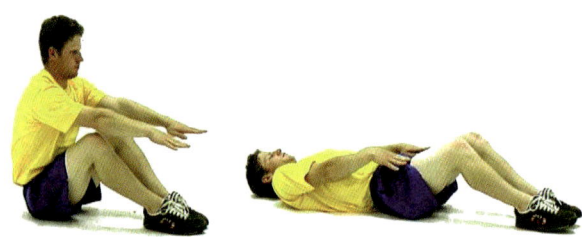

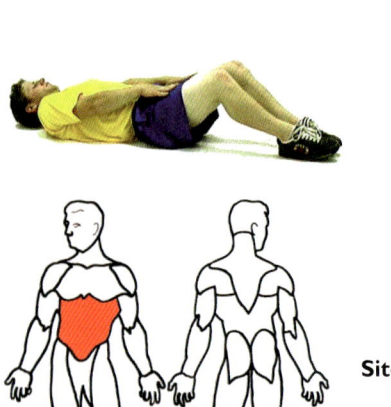

Sit-up.

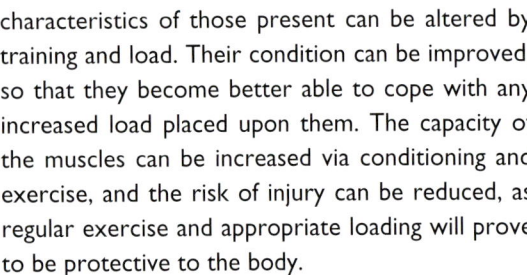

characteristics of those present can be altered by training and load. Their condition can be improved, so that they become better able to cope with any increased load placed upon them. The capacity of the muscles can be increased via conditioning and exercise, and the risk of injury can be reduced, as regular exercise and appropriate loading will prove to be protective to the body.

Within the movement of the core, the origin and insertion of key muscles is important so we know what muscles may be activated by certain movements, for example, the flexion and extension of the spine. This is important when considering strength training and conditioning. We need to know that we are strengthening the target muscles by specific movements. The key is to ensure that it is not just the big, dominant muscles that perform a movement, but that the smaller, synergistic, control muscles are also doing their job. If the big muscles take over and dominate a movement, that is when muscle imbalances occur and there is a risk of injury, as the smaller muscles 'shut off' and become lazy and inactive.

Consideration of the type of muscle contraction required is important when planning a conditioning programme. An individual's objectives, as well as their training experience or injury status, will all affect any decision to include specific exercises. The muscle action can be manipulated by selecting a particular tempo or speed of movement of the contraction. Sometimes, the contraction needs to be quick and explosive, sometimes it should be more endurance-based and regular, and sometimes you want to encourage the muscle to lengthen while it is under tension or loading. There are three main types of muscle contraction:

- **Isometric**: the muscle is activated, but, instead of being allowed to lengthen or shorten, it is held at a constant length or position and contracted.
- **Concentric**: the muscle shortens as it contracts. For example, a sit-up, from a flat position to a flexed position, causes a concentric contraction of the abdominal muscles.
- **Eccentric**: the opposite of concentric, with the muscle lengthening as it contracts under load or gravity, for example, in the downward phase of a sit-up as you extend and return to the floor or bench. To experience this as eccentric load, the tempo or speed of movement would be slow. It may be 2-1-4, which means a count of 2 to flex upward in the sit-up, a count of 1 at the top end position of the sit-up and a count of 4 in the lowering/extension phase of the sit-up to elicit eccentric demands within the muscles.

Another example of eccentric muscle action would be the Romanian dead lift, in which the barbell is slowly lowered with control as the hamstrings lengthen whilst loaded. Eccentric exercise is more likely to produce delayed onset muscle soreness (DOMS) 24 to 48 hours after the session.

INTRODUCTION: WHAT IS THE CORE? WHY IS IT IMPORTANT?

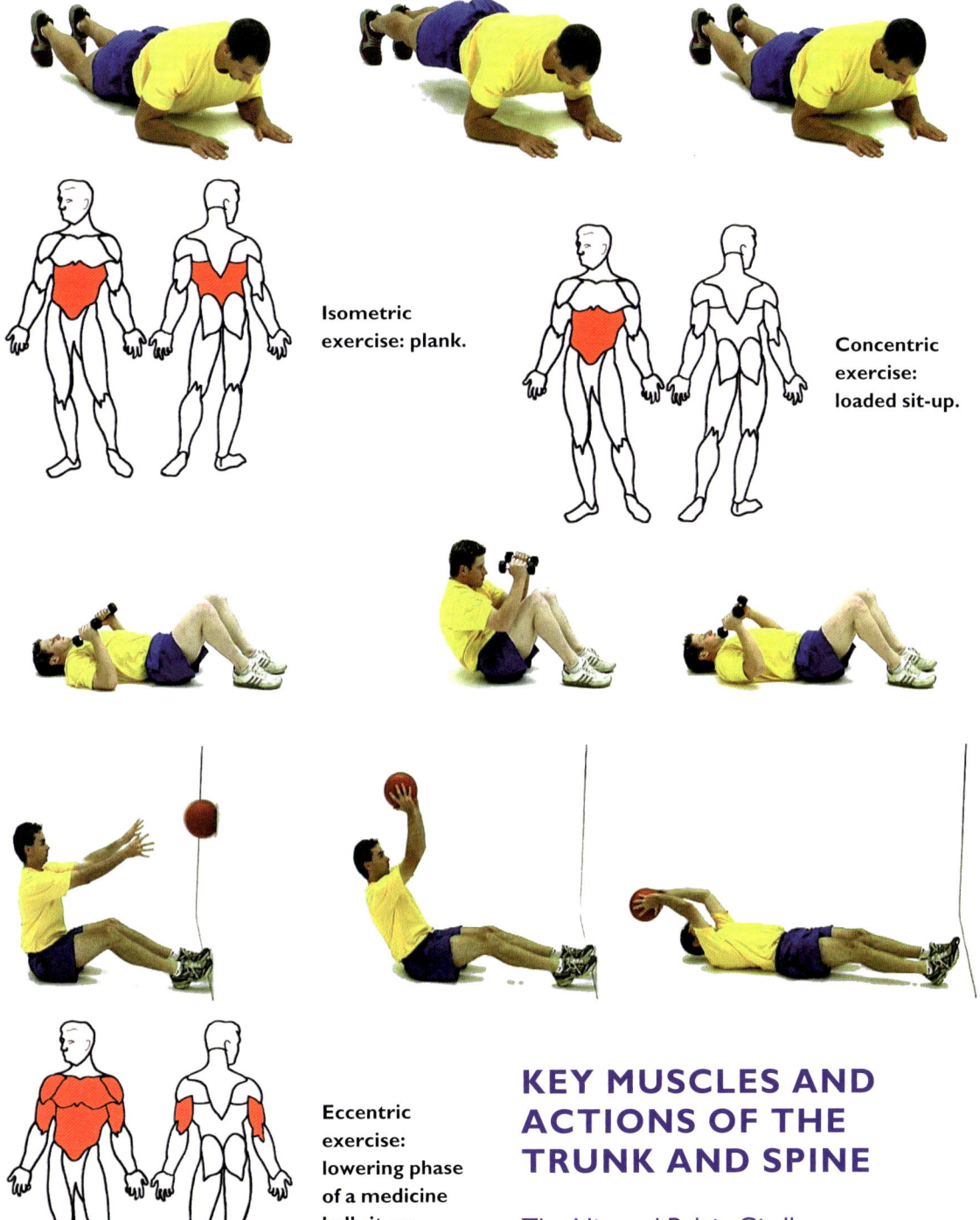

Isometric exercise: plank.

Concentric exercise: loaded sit-up.

Eccentric exercise: lowering phase of a medicine ball sit-up.

KEY MUSCLES AND ACTIONS OF THE TRUNK AND SPINE

The Hip and Pelvic Girdle

These muscles, although predominately in the lower limb, are bi-articular muscles, around the

INTRODUCTION: WHAT IS THE CORE? WHY IS IT IMPORTANT?

Iliopsoas muscles.

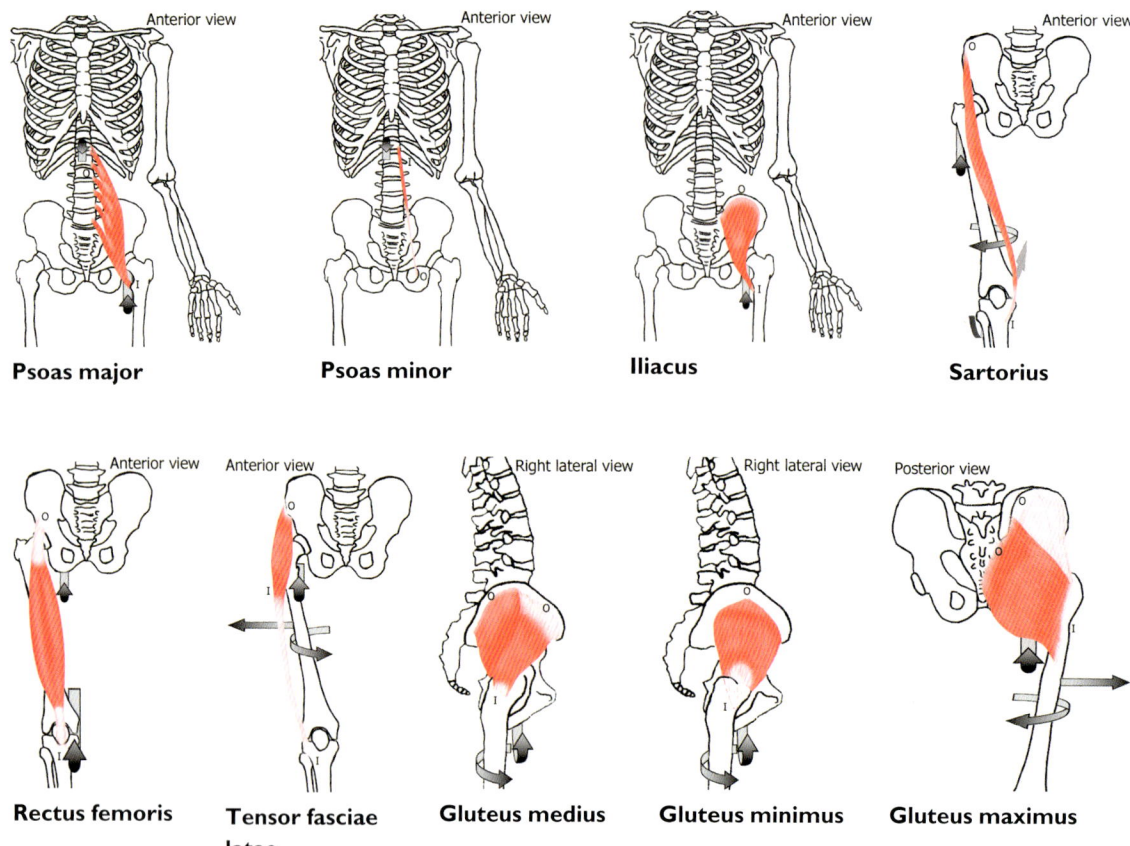

pelvis and hip. Their origin is around the pelvis or lumbar spine and insertion is along the long bone shaft in most cases, so movement will be affected by actions from core activation, pelvic tilt, stability and balance demands, locomotion, movement and function. Looking at the origin (marked 'O' in the images) and insertion (marked 'I' on the images), it is clear why the muscles associated with the hips and pelvic girdle are so involved with spinal stability, and why it is so important to consider these during training and rehabilitation when conditioning the trunk. The arrows indicate the action that the muscle creates when activated – abduction, adduction, rotation, flexion, extension, compression and stabilization.

The Trunk and Spinal Column

This is a very complex system within the body, consisting of twenty-four intricate articulating vertebrae that protect the spinal column with its thirty-one pairs of spinal nerves. The anterior portion of the trunk contains the abdominal muscles, where some sections are linked by fascia rather than bony joints, which adds to its complexity. These intrinsic, stabilizer muscles around the spinal column and trunk are very important in spinal stability and function and need to be trained and stimulated with good activation, functional movement patterns and conditioning.

INTRODUCTION: WHAT IS THE CORE? WHY IS IT IMPORTANT?

Deep lateral rotator muscles.

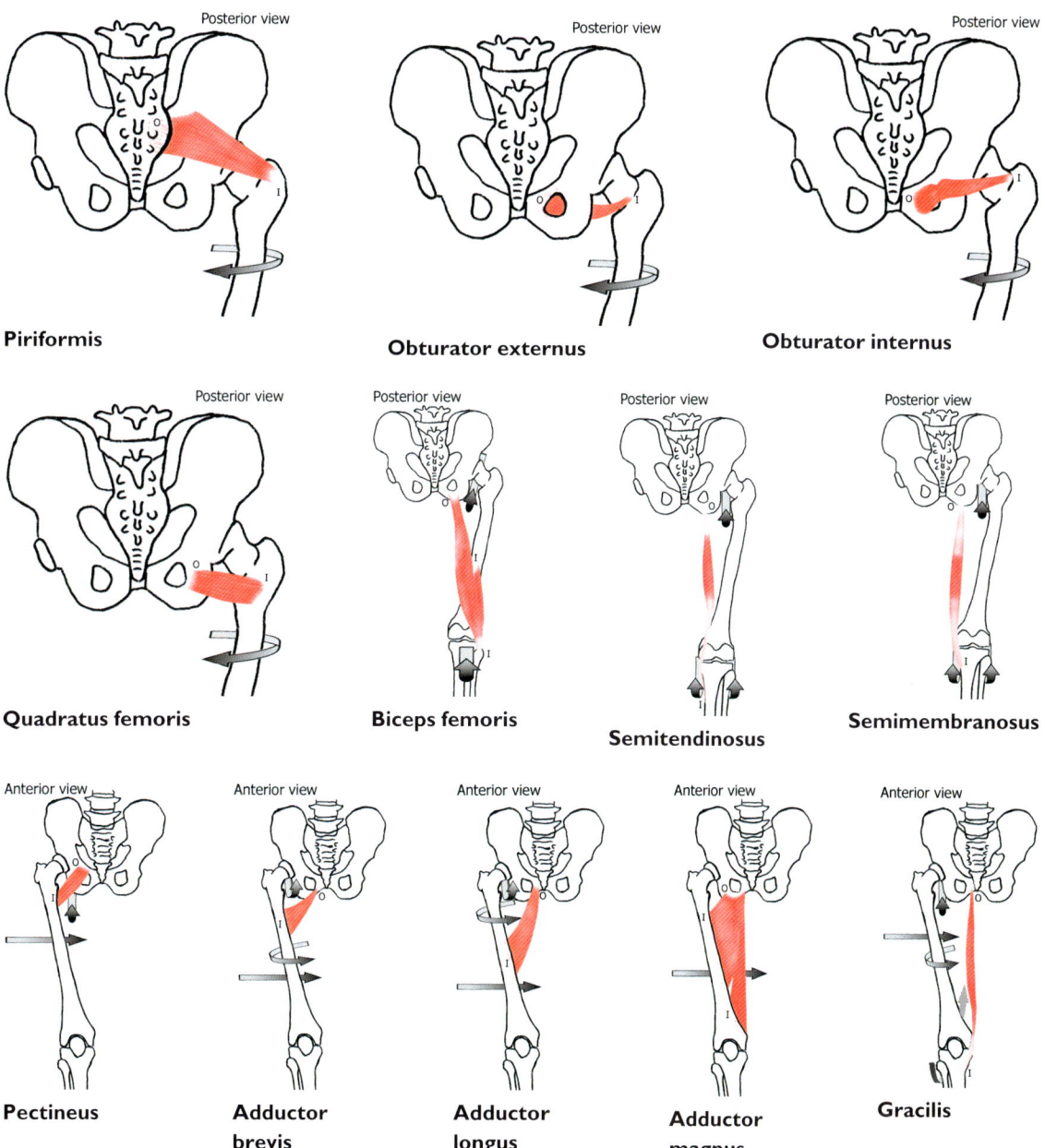

The planes of movement that the spinal column perform are as follows:

- Spinal flexion
- Spinal extension
- Lateral flexion: left or right
- Spinal rotation: left or right

Although there are many muscles around the trunk and spinal column, the main ones involved with core

INTRODUCTION: WHAT IS THE CORE? WHY IS IT IMPORTANT?

strength and stability include, but are not exclusive to, the following:

INNERVATION

The vertebrae and spinal column protect the spinal nerves and associated tissue that innervate the body and its actions. They can be thought of as a protective case surrounding the most precious of cargo. If the nerve fibres become damaged, often this will be permanent and lead to a lack of function or partial or full disability. In normal everyday life, we give little thought to our nervous system and the job that our spinal cord does. But this system is the key to our living: without the feedback to our brain, we would not survive. The brain and spinal cord together make up the central nervous system (CNS). The spinal cord innervates at each level of neural activation to allow for movement around the

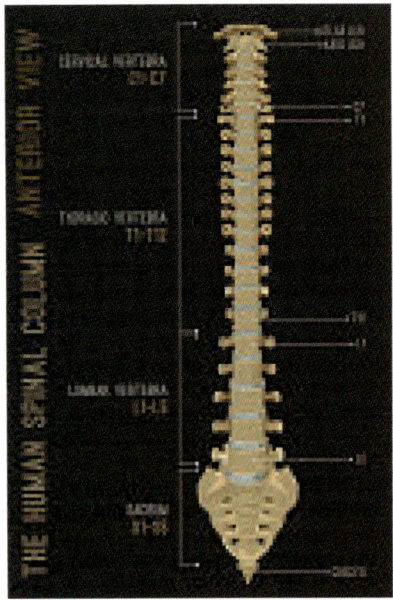

Spinal column: cervical, thoracic and lumbar spine.

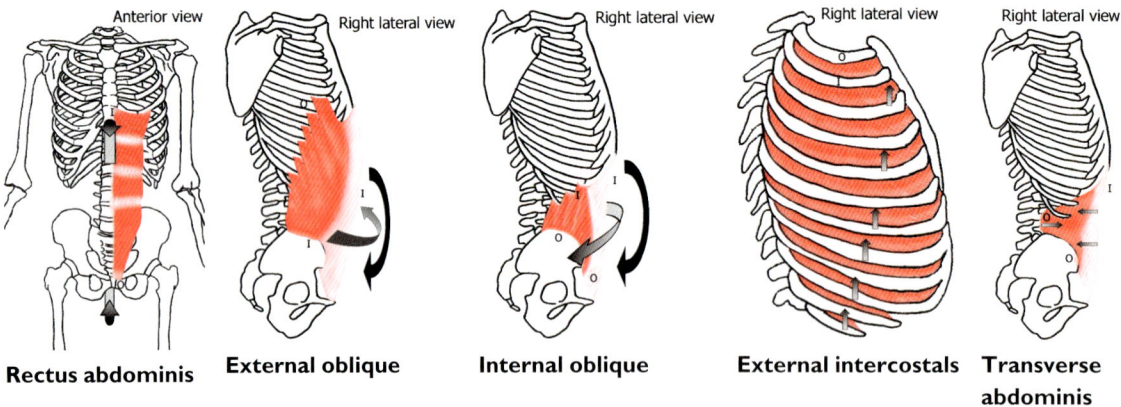

Rectus abdominis — External oblique — Internal oblique — External intercostals — Transverse abdominis

Erector spinae muscles to include:

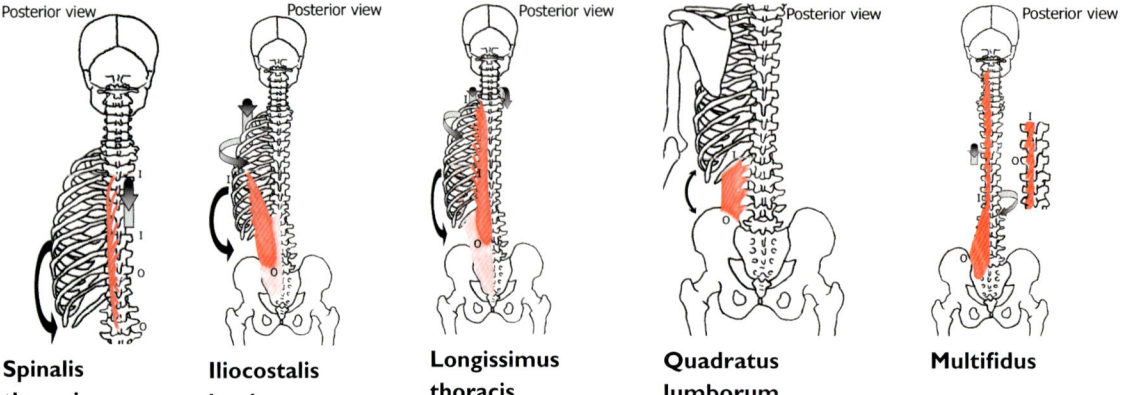

Spinalis thoracis — **Iliocostalis lumborum** — **Longissimus thoracis** — **Quadratus lumborum** — **Multifidus**

INTRODUCTION: WHAT IS THE CORE? WHY IS IT IMPORTANT?

body. The point on the spine that is activated will depend on what muscle or area is innervated and actioned. The main function of the spinal cord is to relay information about what is happening inside and outside the body to and from the brain.

The spinal cord is connected to the rest of the body by thirty-one pairs of spinal nerves, which are part of the peripheral nervous system (PNS). They carry information in the form of nerve impulses from the spinal cord to the rest of the body and from the body to the spinal cord.

Depending on where the spinal nerves branch off, they supply different parts of the body, as follows:

- **Cervical region**: supplies the back of the head, the neck, shoulders, arms, hands and the diaphragm.
- **Thoracic region**: supplies the chest and some parts of the abdomen.
- **Lumbar region**: supplies the lower back as well as parts of the thighs and legs.
- **Sacral region**: supplies the buttocks, most parts of the legs and feet, as well as the anal and genital area (http://www.bbc.co.uk/science/humanbody/body/factfiles/spinalcord/spinal_cord.shtml).

To minimize the risk of spinal injury, the spinal cord is very well protected, surrounded by three tough envelopes called meninges, as well as a clear cerebrospinal fluid that acts as a shock absorber and circulates in the space between the outer and middle meninges and the brain. These are in addition to the vertebral column, which has a hole through the middle of each vertebra that surrounds the spinal cord, the cerebrospinal fluid and the meninges, to aid protection.

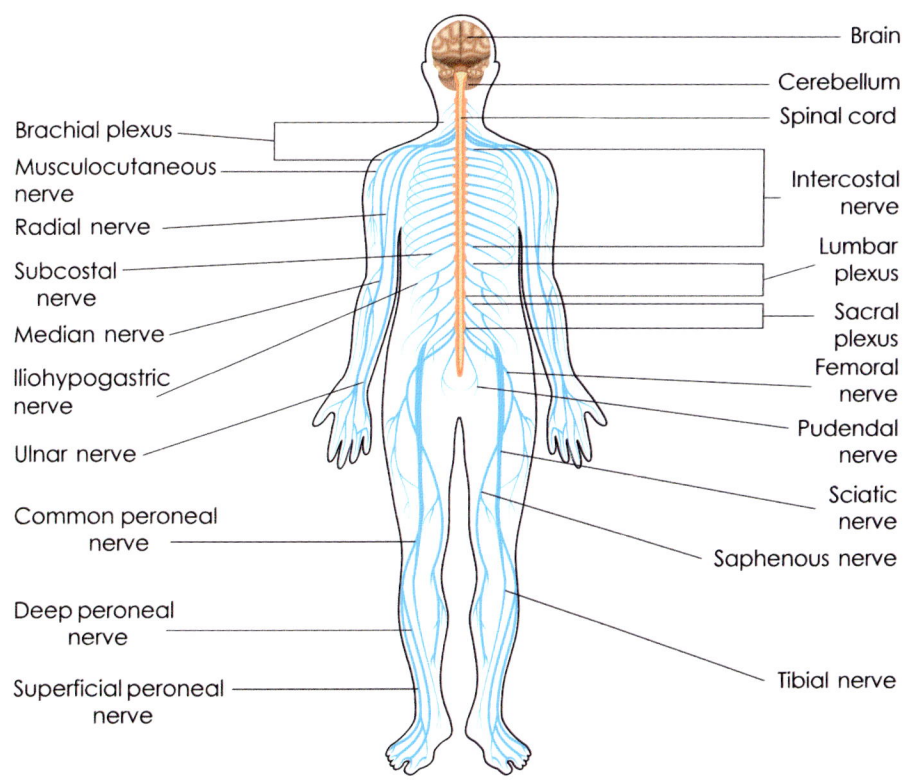

Nervous system.

INTRODUCTION: WHAT IS THE CORE? WHY IS IT IMPORTANT?

MRI SCAN AND RESULTANT REHABILITATION AND PROGRAMMING:

This is an MRI scan (identity removed) on the lumbar spine and the resultant MRI report indicating the findings.

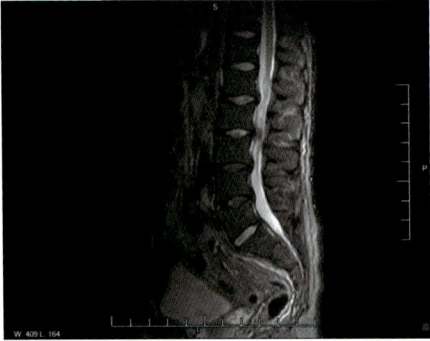

MRI lumbar spine.

Report:

Title: MRI lumbar spine
Clinical indication: Back pain. Right-sided sciatica
Techniques: SagT1/T2 and Axial T2 sequences
Findings:
Normal alignment of the lumbar spine. No vertebral height loss or dislocation demonstrated. Normal bone marrow signal. Normal appearance of the cauda equina.
At L1/L2 level, there is a central disc herniation, resulting in a mild spinal canal stenosis.
At L2/L3 level, there is a central disc protrusion, resulting in a moderate lateral recess calibre stenosis with compression of the descending L3 nerve.
At L3/L4 level, early right paracentral disc herniation noted.
At L4/L5 level, there is a right paracentral disc herniation, resulting in a mild-to-moderate lateral recess stenosis.
At L5/S1 level, there is no significant posterior disc bulge or protrusion identified.
Conclusion:
Changes are more marked at L3–L4 level as described above and may contribute to the patient's symptoms. Further changes also noted at L4–L5 level.

Recommendation:
Clinical correlation is recommended. Spinal surgical referral is advised.

This client was in extreme pain. Everything he did caused discomfort, with a sudden onset after loading. The client is male, in his early forties. He saw his GP after his wife insisted that he got some help and was prescribed muscle relaxants, which managed to break the pain cycle and allowed his body to reduce in spasm, a protective mechanism. Once settled, the client had regular weekly physiotherapy sessions and started a low-level mobility and activation programme. His pain was significant; he could not see the end of the pain cycle or any improvement in function in real time in his mind. This was debilitating and leading to signs of depression.

The client was taking strong muscle relaxants and painkillers as well as non-steroidal anti-inflammatories for a few weeks. It was important that the client was well educated in when to take his medication as much of this type of strong medication is for short-term use only, due to its addictive nature. The prescribed medication and associated indication for use were as follows:

- Naproxen: for pain and inflammation in musculoskeletal disorders
- Co-codamol: for severe pain
- Diazepam: for acute muscle spasm

After regular physiotherapy to help settle the acute phase, the client could begin more functional work again. He plateaued in his recovery for a few weeks with the physiotherapist and was then referred to me. Because of his recent history, his severe pain and his lack of confidence with a return to normal activities, I gave him only three exercises to do, to complement what the physiotherapist had provided. The client was required to complete these three to four times each week and to do them well, with a dedication to excellent movement patterns and technique. I wanted him to believe in and trust the plan and to trust me. The three exercises were as follows:

INTRODUCTION: WHAT IS THE CORE? WHY IS IT IMPORTANT?

Exercise	Sets and repetitions	Rest	Comments/Progressions
Front plank hold	3 x 30 second holds	15–20 seconds	Progress duration as become stronger then leg lift, arm lift, etc.
Double-leg bridging	3 x 8 bridges. 3 second hold at the bridge position. Controlled upward and lowering phase. Tempo: 2-3-2	15–20 seconds	Progress to single leg bridging then bridging on to a Swiss Ball or stability disc.
Supine Swiss ball bridging	3 x 30 second holds	15–20 seconds	Progress to leg lift when stronger and capable. With brace and lift for every duration of hold.

Before the client was referred to me and before he started the specific core work, he was self-selecting to run a few kilometres a week to keep his mind sane, very slowly, after the stress and disappointment of months of inactivity. During the runs he felt uneven in his body and vulnerable, and still had intermittent pain. This quest for normality – completing things that used to be done before pain – is very typical in people who have experienced pain and feel restricted. Even though the client was not quite ready to run physically, he wanted to do it. It was important to him and for his mind, almost as confirmation that he was getting better and recovering. I prescribed the three 'foundation' exercises above and the client was diligent and fully focused in doing them. He was advised to do them three to four times a week, but he probably actually completed them five to six a week, in his enthusiasm and desire to improve.

This provided the client with a sound foundation of strength after the pain, spasm and detraining that followed the sudden onset of low back pain. It was a very positive thing for him to feel and experience. The problem had been life-affecting and now, at last, he was beginning to feel strong and capable again. The foundation core exercises described in this book are very valuable in helping someone through such a journey, from pain to becoming functional and active again. A year on, the client is running again to a good level, completing two or three 10k runs a week, and has progressed to higher-level core-conditioning exercises. His confidence is now so improved that he has signed up to take part in his first-ever marathon. After experiencing at first hand the debilitating nature of low back pain and recognizing the value of a strong core, he has committed to regular core strengthening.

As a strength and conditioning ('S&C') coach, I cannot help but notice that the client's report recommended that, after clinical correlation, 'Spinal surgical referral [would be] advised'. This would surely frighten anyone. It makes me wonder how many people with a similar diagnosis might be referred for surgical intervention when a good, sound, applied core-conditioning programme could prove to be the best solution for them. Of course, compared with invasive spinal surgery, a non-surgical approach and a consequent improvement in strength is definitely going to be the preferred option.

INTRODUCTION: WHAT IS THE CORE? WHY IS IT IMPORTANT?

There are twenty-six vertebrae in the spine in total:

- Cervical (7)
- Thoracic (12)
- Lumbar (5)
- The sacrum, made up of 5 fused vertebrae, and making up the back wall of the pelvis.
- The coccyx, made up of 4 fused vertebrae, an evolutionary remnant of the tail found in most other vertebrates and often called the tailbone.

Considering the innervation from each region of the vertebra within the spine, it is easy to see how a damaged spine, injury, over-use, detraining or chronic bad posture can lead to shooting pains and numbness in the legs or lower limbs, as well as low back pain, which may be the result of a prolapsed disc, for example. Such damage to a disc places pressure on the spinal cord and nerve tissue, which leads to pain and, sometimes, lack of function.

THE KINETIC CHAIN: MOVEMENTS, SLING SYSTEMS AND ACTIVATING THE CORE

When the body moves, high torques and pressures are placed on it and its systems. What supports this load is the strength and capacity of the body as a whole. As the name suggests, the core is an essential component to this balance, synergy and function within the body and this working system.

The kinetic chain is defined as follows by Vern Gambetta, Athletic Development Defining the Discipline, The Gain Network, 2007:

> *The body is a kinetic chain with movement occurring from toenails to fingernails. A sound athletic development program emphasizes integration of all the links of this chain. We must remember that the goal of athletic development is to enhance performance and prevent injury by developing athletes that are completely adaptable to the competitive demands of their sport.*

The concept of an individual's body being completely adaptable to the demands required is relevant not only for athletes, but also for people with physically demanding jobs. Conditioning can prepare a body for that loading and those physical demands. The physical development can make the person adaptable to the demands of, for example, lifting, carrying, twisting and turning, with appropriately conditioned physical parameters at their disposal.

In the concept of the kinetic chain, the joints and segments within the body influence one another during movement. When one joint or muscle is in motion, it creates a chain of events that affects the movement of associated or nearby joints and segments. This is of course relevant in core conditioning and especially when limbs move during core activation.

There are two kinds of kinetic chain exercises: open chain and closed chain. In open kinetic chain exercises, the segment furthest away from the body, known as the distal aspect (usually the hand or foot), is free and not fixed to an object. These exercises involve unrestricted movements in the space of a peripheral segment of the body. A medicine ball rotation is one example of an open chain exercise.

In a closed chain exercise, the distal segment meets with external resistance and remains fixed. Bridging is an example of a closed chain exercise, as the body is in contact with the floor. Closed kinetic chain exercises are more functionally based than open chain exercises (https://medical-dictionary.thefreedictionary.com/kinetic+chain+exercise).

In the case studies within this book, there is a progression from early-phase conditioning or reconditioning. In the rehabilitation-based case studies, this progression is from isometric prone or supine mat- or floor-based work to more challenging and functional core exercises. The next stage involves more dynamic activities in standing, using bands, cables, medicine balls or weight plates with rotation or extension-flexion, either at the legs or arms, to add functional demands. Sometimes, the limbs will hold steady and not move but the core will move as in a core flexion or extension exercise, and sometimes the core will remain braced and the arms or legs will be moving. This concept uses both closed chain and open chain movements. These are all very functional movements, and the effective progression allows for extremely applied movement patterns that are very much transferrable to sport, work demands and activity. This is the body working as a whole unit during these movements and actions, not in isolation.

Taking a mixed martial arts fighter as an example, their capacity to load with a limb extended, on one leg and receiving force back with full contact is impressive. Any weak link in their kinetic chain would be quickly exposed and the athlete would not be capable of performing at the highest level, which would make them vulnerable to injury. The athlete needs to be remarkably robust and strong to cope with external loading and force, at the same time trying to create force against their competitor, often while moving around or on one leg. This strength and capacity comes from the core and demonstrates the kinetic chain and sling systems at work, so functional training and loading through all of these planes of movement and systems are important.

The Sling System

The core musculature is made up of the lumbo-pelvic hip region and involves a number of important muscles:

- Rectus abdominis
- Transversus abdominis
- External oblique
- Internal oblique
- Multifidus
- Erector spinae muscles
- Hip flexors
- Hip adductors
- Glutes
- Pelvic floor muscles

The effectiveness of these muscles working dynamically together will support the body as a whole, especially when it performs complex movements, such as changing direction in any sport, bowling in cricket, playing basketball or playing tennis. All have a requirement for quick feet, agility, mobility and strength throughout the range of movement. The demands placed upon the core in these examples are very high, and if there is a weak spot then injury – a groin strain, hamstring strain, low back pain, or pelvic pain – may occur. The solution to many of these injury problems is to ensure that the athlete or individual has a strong, high-functioning core and associated musculature, as defined by Vern Gambetta above.

This system of muscles is essentially an integrated sling system, like an X across the body, merging around the lumbo-pelvic region. It comprises several muscles that produce force across the body in, as the name suggests, a sling formation. The sling systems are made up as follows:

- **Anterior oblique system**: external and internal oblique with the opposing leg's adductors and intervening anterior abdominal fascia.
- **Posterior oblique system**: the latissimus dorsi and opposing glute maximus.
- **Deep longitudinal system**: erectors, the innervating fascia and biceps femoris.
- **Lateral system**: glute medius and minimus and the opposing adductors of the thigh.

A muscle may participate in more than one sling and the slings may overlap and interconnect, depending on the demands being placed on the body. The hypothesis is that the slings have no beginning or end but rather connect to assist in the

INTRODUCTION: WHAT IS THE CORE? WHY IS IT IMPORTANT?

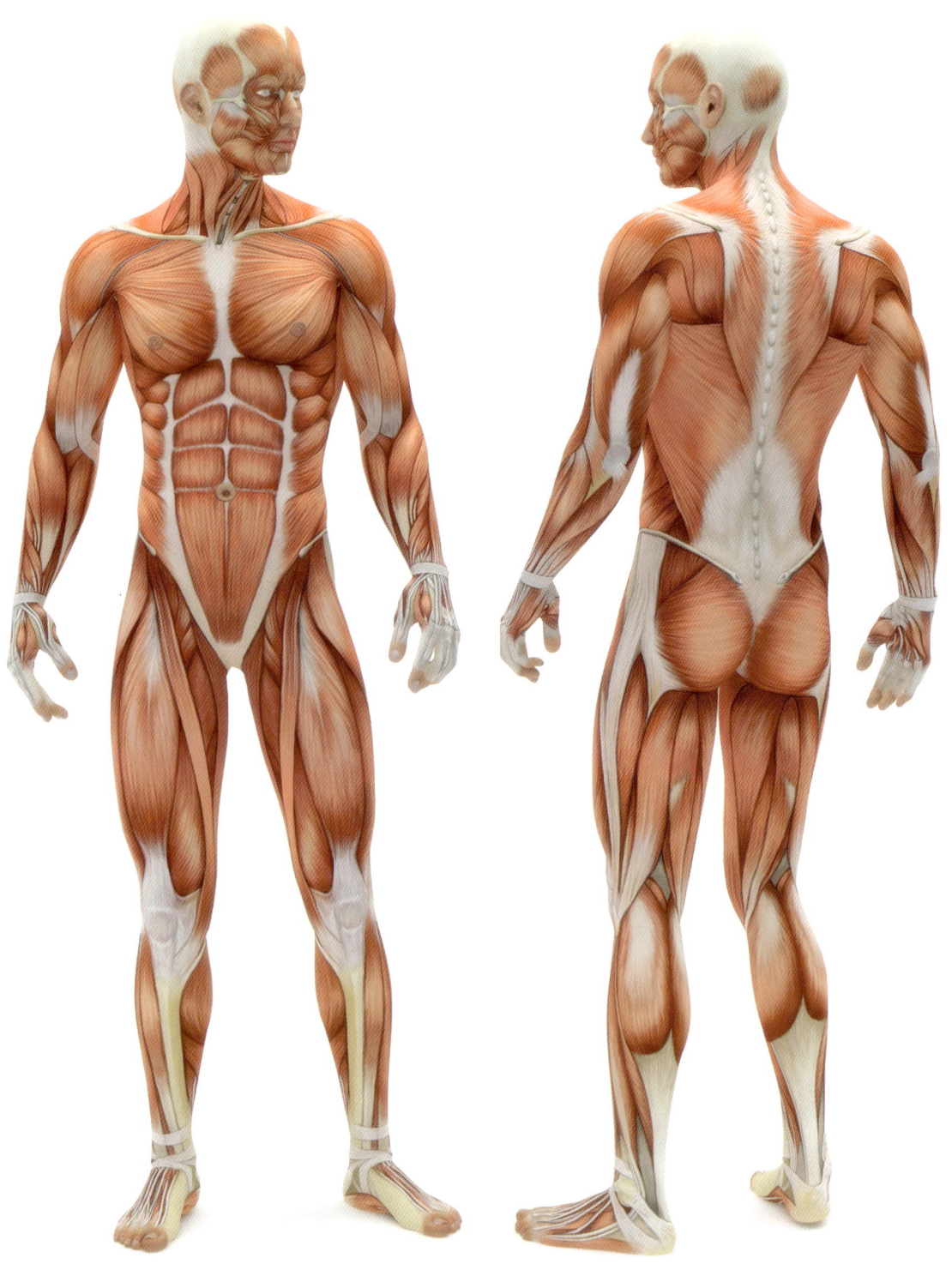

Lumbo-pelvic hip region/core musculature on the human body.

INTRODUCTION: WHAT IS THE CORE? WHY IS IT IMPORTANT?

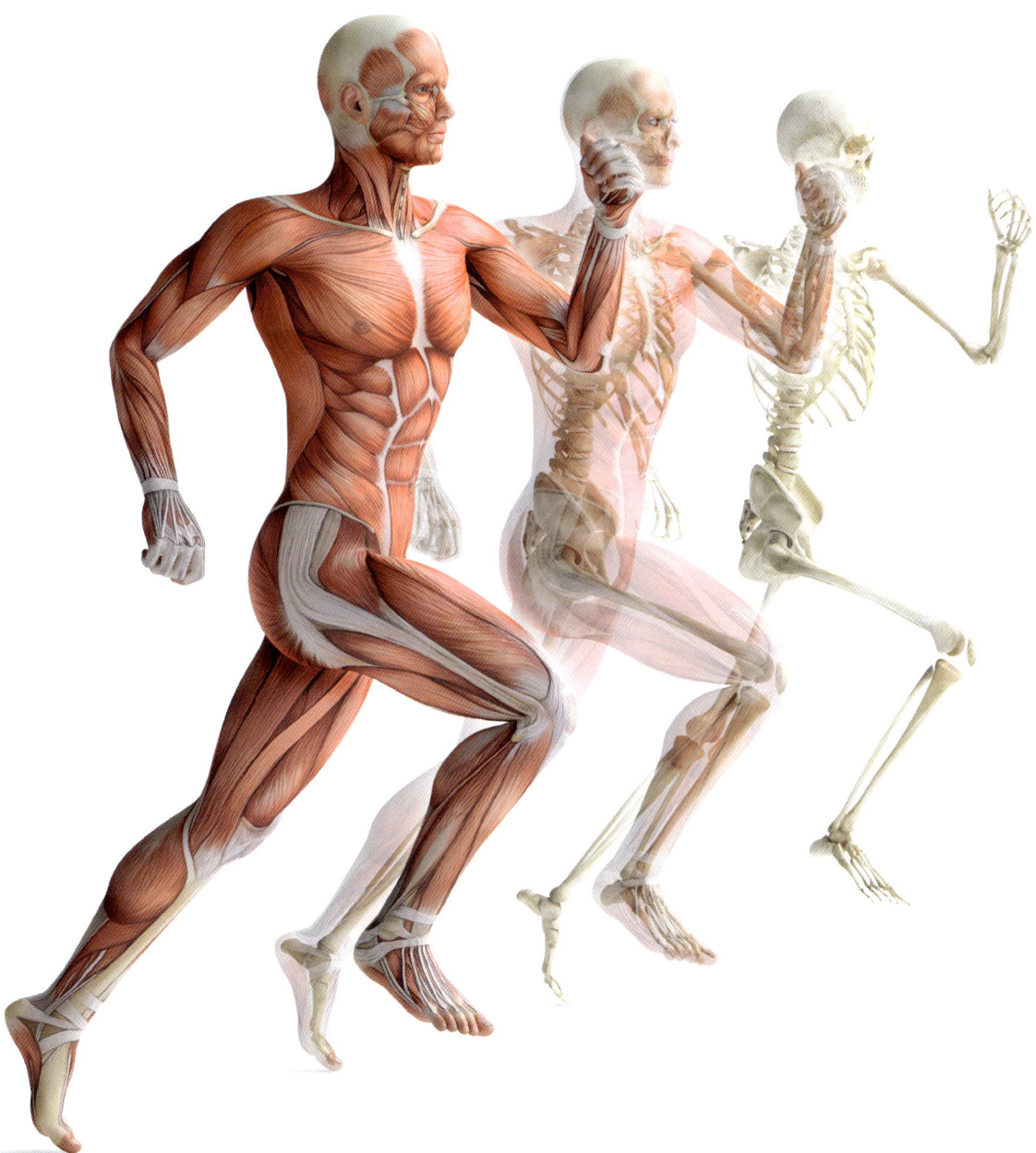

The human body showing the musculature of the sling systems.

transference of forces through the body. It is possible that the slings are all part of one interconnected myofascial system and the particular sling (anterior oblique, posterior oblique, lateral system, deep longitudinal system), which is identified during any motion, is merely due to the activation of selective parts of the whole sling during its activation and movement.

The Serape Effect

The serape effect, similar to the sling systems, is a way to rotationally train the core, as discussed by Juan Carlos Santana, MEd, CSCS (National Strength and Conditioning Association, *Journal of Strength and Conditioning* Volume 25, Number 2, pages 73–74, 2003). He describes the function of the serape effect as follows:

> *The purpose of the serape effect is to provide the muscles of the core an optimal length-tension environment for maximum force production. The serape effect is the result of the interaction of four pairs of muscles: the rhomboids, the serratus anterior, the external obliques, and the internal obliques… To strengthen the serape musculature, we use several approaches. When appropriate, we certainly use traditional exercises to strengthen the entire body. These include the Olympic-style lifts and traditional strength lifts such as squats, bench presses and pull-ups. However, since the serape muscles are usually used standing and involve rotation, we also include training that provides loading capabilities to this environment.*

The serape effect is a rotational trunk movement that involves ballistic motions, such as those seen in throwing or kicking. It stretches these muscles to their greatest length in order to create a snap-back effect. When this tension is released from these muscles, they shorten for the completion of the movement, and a greater velocity is applied than would have been the case had the muscles performed from a normal resting length (https://en.wikipedia.org/wiki/Serape_effect).

Strengthening the Posterior Chain

The posterior chain is another area that requires attention to ensure overall core and body strength. It includes the biceps femoris, gluteus maximus, erector spinae muscle group, trapezius, and posterior deltoids. The core strength is particularly influenced by the biceps femoris, gluteus maximus and erector spinae muscles from the posterior chain. If these are weak and poorly conditioned, then the function of the sling systems and the serape effect will be compromised. Postural control will be poor and having a weak posterior chain can also affect other parts of the body. For example, an individual may have knee pain, Achilles problems or plantar fasciitis, but often the area of pain will not necessarily be the cause of the problem or the area of weakness. It is sometimes necessary to look up the chain in the body and be a little more holistic in any review and assessment of the problem

In some cases, my clients with lower limb pain have a very weak posterior chain, with weak glutes, hamstrings and low back. Strengthening their posterior chain tends to off-load the physical demands through the kinetic chain and can often solve the initial problem. Clients with Achilles problems or plantar fasciitis, for example, have often experienced a positive outcome using this whole-body strategy and awareness. Again, this is an example of the body working globally and identifies the ways in which a weak link can affect the chain, pain and function.

Trunk Muscle Coordination

Clearly, the sling systems and the posterior chain are all important contributors to strengthening the core, but Hodges and Richardson (1999) also focused on the role of transversus abdominis in healthy individuals and the response of this muscle in patients with low back pain. They wanted to compare trunk muscle coordination in people with and without low back pain with varying speeds of limb movement. Abdominal and back extensor muscle activity in association with upper limb movement was compared among three speeds of movement and between people with and without low back pain. On each participant, the onset of electromyographic activity of the trunk and limb muscles, frequency of trunk muscle responses, and angular velocity of arm movements were measured. They concluded from their sample of fourteen participants with low back pain and fourteen without low back pain (N = 28) that early activation of transversus abdominis and obliquus internus abdominis occurred in the majority of trials, with movement at both the fast and intermediate speeds for the control group (those with no low back pain). In contrast, subjects with low back pain failed to recruit their transversus abdominis or obliquus internus abdominis in advance of fast limb movement, and no activity of the abdominal muscles was recorded in the majority of intermediate speed trials. In these trials there was no difference between groups for slow movement, with both the control group (no low back pain) and the low back pain group responding to the movement at a slow speed. These results indicate that the mechanism of preparatory spinal control is altered in people with lower back pain for movement at a variety of speeds (Hodges and Richardson, 1999).

Similarly, Silfies *et al.* (2009) investigated alterations in trunk muscle timing patterns in subgroups of patients with mechanical low back pain and a control group. They also found that the activation timing patterns and number of muscles functioning in feedforward were statistically different between the patients with mechanical low back pain and the control group. The control group activated the external oblique, lumbar multifidus and erector spinae muscles in a feedforward manner, but mechanical low back pain subgroups demonstrated significantly different timing patterns and delay, much as they did in the research carried out by Hodges and Richardson.

Activating the Core

This supports the theory that at a low-level requirement most people can subconsciously activate their core musculature to provide the spinal support and strength that they need as they move. However, as these movements become more demanding, quicker or more complex, or if the person is in a state of low back pain, the muscle activation may be inhibited, which in turn will make the body more susceptible to injury. Consciously, and then subconsciously, activating the lumbo-pelvic musculature effectively appears to be protective in the management of low back pain and compromised in those with low back pain.

This research demonstrated that the transversus abdominis, external oblique, lumbar multifidus and erector spinae muscles are anticipatory muscles for stabilization of the lower back and are recruited prior to the initiation of any movement of the upper or lower extremity – if things are working well. The research also showed that this anticipatory recruitment is absent or may be delayed in patients with low back pain. This leads to the hypothesis that, in a person with low back pain, there may be a delayed firing of the lumbo-pelvic muscles. Consequently, training and conditioning these muscles and making them stronger and more responsive should protect the spine better, and reduce the incidence of low back pain. This would also make sense with pain inhibition and resultant injury: if an individual is in pain and these muscles are not activating as a result, then further injury may be more likely.

Research conducted by Moseley *et al.* (2002) sought to determine the activity of the deep and superficial fibres of the lumbar multifidus during voluntary movement of the arm. The multifidus contributes to the stability of the lumbar spine. Because the deep and superficial parts of the multifidus are near the centre of lumbar joint rotation, the superficial fibres are well suited to control spine orientation, and the deep fibres to control intervertebral movement. The goal of the research was to determine if this was accurate. With the analysis of electromyographic activity, which was recorded in both the deep and superficial multifidus, transversus abdominis, erector spinae and deltoid using selective intramuscular electrodes and surface electrodes during single and repetitive arm movements, this was established. The latency of electromyographic onset in each muscle during single movements and the pattern of electromyographic activity during repetitive movements was compared between muscles. The researchers concluded that the deep and superficial fibres of the multifidus are differentially active during single and repetitive movements of the arm. The data from this study support the hypothesis that the superficial multifidus contributes to the control of spine orientation, and that the deep multifidus has a role in controlling intersegmental motion (Moseley, Hodges and Gandevia, 2002).

BREATHING AND BRACING

Nelson (2012) discusses the importance of effective diaphragmatic breathing and how this can affect spinal health, and how insufficient and uncoordinated diaphragm activation can compromise the stability of the spine. In her opinion, intra-abdominal pressure is very important in protecting the spine when lifting heavy weights in the gym, or when lifting at home or for work. The technique includes a slight breath outwards, hold and brace during the lifting phase, to provide intra-abdominal pressure around the spine, almost like a girdle. It is important to coach the individual not to hold their breath, like the Valsalva manoeuvre, but to brace and breathe, in order to protect the spine.

The concept of bracing is raised by Grenier and McGill (2007), who looked at the comparison between hollowing and bracing via EMG analysis with eight subjects. The study assessed the influence of different abdominal activation strategies on mechanical stability in the lumbar spine, specifically the hollowing technique and the bracing technique. Despite the small sample in the study, they found that the brace technique improved stability of the spine by 32 per cent. There seems to be no mechanical rationale for using an abdominal hollow, or the transversus abdominis alone, to enhance stability. Indeed, research by Richardson *et al.* (2002) states that the transversus abdominis may be activated independently of other abdominal muscles at very low levels of challenge, at around 1–2 per cent of maximum voluntary contraction. However, at higher levels of activation, when people perform tasks requiring spine stability, the transversus abdominis has also been shown to be a synergist of the internal oblique so it does not work in isolation. Bracing creates patterns that better enhance stability based upon higher spinal demands.

My personal coaching cues include a focus on both hollowing or drawing in and a brace. I think people like to feel the sensation of the brace as they contract through the core, where things feel strong and tightened, but, due to exposure to activities such as Pilates they are often more familiar with the hollowing-in technique as described by Fredericson and Moore (2005). An improved spinal stability, as evidenced with bracing of 32 per cent when compared to hollowing, is certainly significant and should be considered when coaching and training the core.

USING LOADS IN TRAINING

Because the muscles of the trunk and torso stabilize the spine from the pelvis to the neck and shoulder via the sling systems, they allow the transfer of powerful movements of the arms and legs. All powerful movements originate from the centre of the body out, and never from the limbs alone. If you stand upright and try to lift something heavy purely with your arms, it may be difficult. However, if you add in bent knees and a strong braced core and back, a lower centre of gravity and a larger base of support, you can create more force and lift much heavier or more easily. This is the body working efficiently.

Overhead training or loaded carries have been shown to help develop core strength when included within applied functional training. The application of core training in standing or whilst moving is perhaps a little unfamiliar for regular core strength conditioning, being less traditional than the typical floor-based core exercises often prescribed for motor learning, activation and control. These foundation core exercises do have a very important role to play, especially in rehabilitation and early levels of core conditioning. However, as an individual progresses and becomes stronger, the demands placed upon them by their conditioning coach need to become more applied, functional and challenging, to match the demands that they face in their daily living, activities or sport.

Rusin and Butcher (2017) discuss the benefit of loaded carries with a number of variations as a great way to challenge and develop more functional core conditioning for an athlete. They suggest that, while direct and isolated core activation methods play a role in the care of injured athletes, in order to adequately challenge core stability, the strength and conditioning coach can create high levels of neurological demand. Often this means attempting to enhance core control in standing positions through common movements, such as walking. This is where the inclusion of loaded carries can be a viable option. (Rusin and Butcher, 2017) Loading during each phase of walking, including the stance and swing phases in both legs, provides a suitable opportunity to tap into creating torque and tension throughout the entire body. The added load also acts as a destabilizing force, resulting in the need to maintain walking posture throughout the carry.

Rusin and Butcher (2017) highlight the benefit of using kettlebells or dumbbells held on either side of the body, placed high or low, and walking for varying time durations with a certain percentage of body weight load. The load will depend on the requirements of the individual – rehabilitation, general fitness or elite sporting performance. The authors also suggest holding one kettlebell overhead and one by the side, for example, to challenge the core and control. Asymmetric work as described by McGill (2010) uniquely challenges the lateral musculature (quadratus lumborum and oblique abdominal wall) in a way that is not possible with a bilateral symmetrical squat, for example. This type of asymmetrical loading challenges the body and creates an ability for any person who runs and cuts, carries a load, and so on, to strengthen in a slightly different way. Such a challenge is always good for high-performance athletes and to introduce stimulation to training.

This a great way to train and places functional demands on the athlete. It teaches them how to move with load and to be efficient. Of course, when the load is removed in competition, the hope is that the athlete has developed and transferred the training stimulus into effective performance.

The concept of disturbance training with the core is an effective progression: using chaos to condition! Different weighted dumbbells or kettle bells, different weight plates on the end of a barbell, water-based containers that swill around as they are lifted and carried, or sand bags, BOSU or balance beams, are all ways to add disturbance to more high-end activities. Resistance bands, ropes and partner-based work, pulling and pushing as you brace and complete the movement against a partner, will all add to the challenge and functional work capacity for the athlete.

COORDINATION AND STABILITY

In relation to running, Fredericson and Moore (2005) found that any weakness or lack of sufficient coordination in core musculature can lead to less efficient movements, compensatory movement patterns, strain, over-use and injury. This research recommends that, for middle- and long-distance runners, whose events involve balanced and powerful movements of the body propelling itself forward and catching itself in complex motor patterns, a strong foundation of muscular balance is essential. They state that the purpose of basic core stabilization exercises is not only to increase stability, but also, more importantly, to gain coordination and timing of the deep abdominal-wall musculature.

It is extremely important to do the basic exercises correctly as they are the foundation of all other core exercises and movement patterns. These basic exercises emphasize maintaining the lumbar spine in a neutral position (which is the mid-range position between lumbar extension and flexion), allowing for the natural curvature of the spine. This first stage of core stability training begins with the athlete learning to stabilize the abdominal wall. Proper activation of these muscles is considered crucial in the first stages of a core stability programme, before progressing to more dynamic and multi-planar activities.

Kavcic *et al.* (2004) completed a systematic biomechanical analysis involving an artificial perturbation applied to individual lumbar muscles to assess their potential stabilizing role. They wanted to identify which torso muscles stabilize the spine during different loading conditions and to identify possible mechanisms of function. Spine kinematics, external forces, and fourteen channels of torso electromyography were recorded for seven stabilization exercises in order to capture the individual motor control strategies adopted by different people. They concluded from this research that no single muscle dominated in the enhancement of spine stability, and their individual roles were continuously changing across tasks. Clinically, if the goal is to train for stability, enhancing motor patterns that incorporate many muscles rather than targeting just a few is justifiable.

This is contrary to the belief of Hodges and Richardson (1999), which is greatly in favour of transversus abdominis activation and hollowing to activate. Kavcic's research cited above is also in line with McGill (2010), who raises the point that it is not just transversus abdominis that is important for core stabilization and that all of the lumbo-pelvic muscles are drawn into action at different times, based upon the loading pattern through the body. McGill (2010) canvases that there is evidence suggesting that a strong core allows strength to radiate out peripherally to more distant regions of the body, which of course improves function and will be protective, based around injury risk. He goes on to discuss that true spinal stability is achieved with what he terms 'balanced' stiffening from the entire musculature around the spine, including the rectus abdominis and the abdominal wall; quadratus lumborum; latissimus dorsi; and the back extensors of longissimus, iliocostalis and multifidus. In his opinion, focusing on a single muscle generally does not enhance stability but creates patterns that, when quantified, result in less stability.

Isometric core stability training begins with learning to co-contract and brace the lumbo-pelvic hip muscles effectively. This has been identified by a number of research papers as being key to the lumbar-support mechanism. Learning to activate these muscles effectively will ensure that the core is stimulated, which will allow for strength development and protect the lumbar spine and pelvic region. The core needs to be rigid and robust, yet also mobile and supportive, to allow locomotion and movement.

The core, lumbo-pelvic hip region, posterior chain and sling systems are complex structures that work together and not in isolation within the body. They serve to protect the spine and create

INTRODUCTION: WHAT IS THE CORE? WHY IS IT IMPORTANT?

efficiency of movement. An understanding of how these coordinate and lead to proficiency of movement and a stronger spinal support system is important when prescribing an effective core conditioning programme.

Based upon the research and the protective role that the lumbo-pelvic hip and spinal muscles perform, the concept of balanced stiffness as discussed by McGill appears to be the most effective strategy for activation, training and conditioning this region. Using appropriate cues to coach and understand the movement patterns is important and will lead to positive outcomes and improved core activation, strength and function.

CHAPTER 2

MUSCULOSKELETAL DISORDERS: THE FINANCIAL COST AND POSSIBLE SOLUTIONS

If becoming stronger means that an individual's risk of low back pain will be reduced, then how strong does that individual need to be? Is it just a little stronger and a little more activated? Or is it purely being fit for purpose? If your job or daily demands require good core strength, then surely being fit for purpose, and being able to identify what that is, is what counts. Maybe no one knows specifically how strong anyone should be, but certainly the incidence of low back pain and associated injury in the general population indicates that that population does need to be stronger.

If someone is clinically pain-free with no spinal symptoms, does that mean that their risk of low back pain or injury is reduced? Should they still address their levels of strength, despite being asymptomatic? Or are functional tests the best way to actually assess our risk of low back injury? Many people who have a sudden onset of low back pain have no signs or symptoms before an acute event, yet, if everyone over a certain age was scanned, it is likely that there would be evidence of wear and tear, indicating a possible increased risk of injury and the resultant onset of pain. Surely taking a proactive approach to back health and ensuring a certain level of strength is a good idea, considering the incidence and debilitating nature of sudden-onset back pain. As the population ages, the incidence of low back pain appears to increase.

There are three main musculoskeletal changes reported in the literature as individuals age that need to be considered and lead to an increased risk of injury:

- Reduction in joint mobility.
- Decrease in muscular strength.
- Slowing of reaction and movement times.

THE STATISTICS: RISK AND FINANCIAL COST

The Health and Safety Executive Work-Related Musculoskeletal Disorders (WRMSDs) Statistics in Great Britain 2017 indicate that males over 35 years old had an increased incidence of low back pain consistent from the over 35-year category all the way to over-55s. In females there is a similar trend, with under 35-year-olds experiencing the least amount of low back pain, but, unlike the men, who have a consistent risk over 35 years old, in females this risk increases again in the 45- to 54-year-olds and again in the over-55s, having statistically significantly higher rates of low back pain progressively increasing as the female age group becomes older.

According to the same statistics, the rate of self-reported work-related musculoskeletal disorders mainly affecting the back shows a generally downward trend from the past. In 2016–17, the prevalence rate was 590 cases per 100,000 workers. This equates to 194,000 total cases in 2016–17, which is 38 per cent of all work-related musculoskeletal disorders. In 2016–17, the number of working days lost due to work-related back disorders was 3.2 million, with an average number of days lost per case of 16.5. There has been a downward trend as work safety has improved over the past ten years or so, with a plateau of these figures occurring since 2010–11. Despite the downward trend, however, there is no disputing that the issue costs businesses millions in lost time and working hours.

The costs to Britain according to the Health and Safety at Work summary statistics for Great Britain 2017 are as follows:

- Total costs showed a downward trend between 2004–05 and 2009–10: this fall was driven by a reduction in the number of workplace injuries. Since then, the annual cost has been broadly level.
- Total costs include both financial and human costs. Financial costs cover loss of output, health care and other payments made. Human costs are the monetary valuation given to pain, grief, suffering and loss of life.
- The total costs of work-related injury and ill health (excluding long-latency illness such as cancer) in 2015–16 were £14.9 billion.
- Of the £14.9 billion, £9.7 billion represented the annual costs of new cases of work-related ill health in 2015–16, excluding long-latency illness such as cancer.
- The total annual costs of workplace injury in 2015–16 were £5.3 billion.

(Estimates based on Labour Force Survey and RIDDOR for 2014–15 and 2016–17, and HSE Costs to Britain Model. © Crown Copyright 2017. Published by the Health and Safety Executive November 2017. *Contains public sector information licensed under the Open Government Licence v3.0.*)

The above monetary values and costs represent all work-related injury and illness, to include work-related musculoskeletal disorders, occupational lung disease, workplace injury, work-related stress, depression and anxiety, and work-related ill health. Although these values have decreased and now have appeared to have plateaued over the past few years, as a result of health and safety awareness and education, better and safer equipment and more employee and employer awareness, there is no question that the costs to business, and also to the individual and their family, are significant.

The sudden onset of low back pain can be life-affecting. Heavy lifting and carrying remain the primary drivers for low back pain at work within the construction and health/social industries. However, in recent years, the poor posture and repetitive movements of keyboard users account for around 12 per cent of musculoskeletal disorders, including low back pain. Perhaps, addressing the three key areas of risk in low back injury in older populations – a reduction in joint mobility, a decrease in muscular strength and the slowing of reaction and movement times – could reduce the incidence of injury and avoid the personal cost to the individual and the financial cost to all involved.

An appropriate applied strength and conditioning programme, aimed at addressing these three key areas, could therefore be a valuable addition to a workplace wellness programme. It could also contribute to any individual's self-preservation as they progress through their career and life.

MUSCULAR IMBALANCES AND ASSESSMENT: PATIENT QUESTIONNAIRES, CLINICAL ASSESSMENT AND MUSCULAR TESTING

The study of the relationship between workers and their environment, especially the equipment they use, is called ergonomics or biotechnology (*Collins English Dictionary – Complete and Unabridged*, 10th Edition). It is about the applied science of equipment design, for the workplace, intended to maximize productivity by reducing operator fatigue and discomfort.

An ergonomic specialist may attend a place of work and complete a workplace assessment to ensure that the employees' lifting technique is appropriate and low risk, or that they have appropriate equipment to help them do the job at hand. For example, a number of years ago, employees of the Royal Mail would routinely carry a heavy post bag on their delivery rounds, inevitably increasing their risk of postural issues, back pain and movement challenges. In recent years, the company has introduced a front-pushing postal trolley, to reduce the risk of injury for staff. This is a good example of a modification leading to better safety standards and a reduction in the incidence of injury.

Although it is largely beyond the scope of this book, and is not strictly speaking part of the role of the S&C coach, it is important to consider the process of assessment in cases of low back pain, and how this can be managed. A good chartered physiotherapist, athletic trainer or General Practitioner will be able to conduct an effective subjective and objective clinical assessment to establish the cause of any symptoms, and put an appropriate plan in place. All practitioners will have their own procedure and 'red flags' to identify when assessing someone with low back pain, but in summary diagnosis can be established as follows:

- The patient is classified according to the diagnostic triage recommended in international back pain guidelines (Koes *et al.*, 2010). Serious causes of back pain include fracture, cancer, infection and ankylosing spondylitis. Specific causes may be related to neurological deficits, such as radiculopathy, caudal equina syndrome. Serious conditions are rare and account for 1–2 per cent of people presenting with low back pain. 5–10 per cent present with specific causes of low back pain with neurological deficits, but it is important to screen for these conditions (Henschke *et al.*, 2009).
- When serious and specific causes of low back pain have been ruled out, individuals are said to have non-specific (or simple or mechanical) back pain.
- Non-specific low back pain accounts for over 90 per cent of patients presenting to primary care (Koes *et al.*, 2006).

Initially, a thorough patient history will be taken. Areas of importance include age, occupation, mechanism of injury, how long has the pain been present, is the pain worsening, staying the same, or intermittent? Are there any specific movement patterns or actions that cause the onset of pain? What medication is the patient taking? How is their general health and wellbeing? Is there any anxiety or stress? Has there been a change in lifestyle – for example, a new baby? These are all very important inquisitive questions to help establish some background information before the clinical, objective assessment. Any particular concerns based upon this discussion should be noted by the practitioner.

In addition to the practitioner's note-taking and clinical experience, it is important to pay attention to the verbal and physical cues from a patient as they discuss their issue.

Patient Questionnaires

Other tools to help establish a patient's presentation include patient questionnaires, which may be useful for tracking pain and levels of function. There are many options to choose from, but a few examples include the following:

- The Quebec Back Pain Disability Scale (QBPDS): a 20-item self-administered instrument designed to assess the level of functional disability in individuals with back pain. The Quebec Scale can be recommended as an outcome measure in clinical trials, and for monitoring the progress of individual patients participating in treatment or rehabilitation programmes (Kopec et al., 1995).
- Oswestry Low Back Pain Disability Questionnaire: a patient-completed questionnaire, which gives a subjective percentage score of level of function (disability) in activities of daily living in those rehabilitating from low back pain. It examines perceived level of disability in ten everyday activities of daily living (Fisher and Johnston, 1997).
- Keele STarT Back Screening Tool (SBST): a simple prognostic questionnaire that helps clinicians identify modifiable risk factors (biomedical, psychological and social) for back pain disability. The resulting score stratifies patients into low-, medium- or high-risk categories and for each category there is a matched treatment package. This approach has been shown to reduce back-pain-related disability and to be cost-effective (keele.ac.uk/sbst/startbacktool).
- Roland-Morris Disability Questionnaire (see below): designed to assess self-rated physical disability caused by low back pain. It is most sensitive for patients with mild to moderate disability due to acute, sub-acute or chronic low back pain. The RMDQ is scored by adding up the number of items checked by the patient. The score can therefore vary from 0 to 24. This can be used to track pain and progress.

THE ROLAND-MORRIS DISABILITY QUESTIONNAIRE

When your back hurts, you may find it difficult to do some of the things you normally do.

This list contains sentences that people have used to describe themselves when they have back pain. When you read them, you may find that some stand out because they describe you *today*.

As you read the list, think of yourself *today*. When you read a sentence that describes you today, put a tick against it. If the sentence does not describe you, then leave the space blank and go on to the next one. Remember, only tick the sentence if you are sure it describes you today.

1. I stay at home most of the time because of my back.
2. I change position frequently to try to get my back comfortable.
3. I walk more slowly than usual because of my back.
4. Because of my back I am not doing any of the jobs that I usually do around the house.
5. Because of my back, I use a handrail to get upstairs.
6. Because of my back, I lie down to rest more often.
7. Because of my back, I have to hold on to something to get out of an easy chair.
8. Because of my back, I try to get other people to do things for me.
9. I get dressed more slowly than usual because of my back.
10. I only stand for short periods of time because of my back.
11. Because of my back, I try not to bend or kneel down.
12. I find it difficult to get out of a chair because of my back.
13. My back is painful almost all the time.

(continued)

> 14. I find it difficult to turn over in bed because of my back.
> 15. My appetite is not very good because of my back pain.
> 16. I have trouble putting on my socks (or stockings) because of the pain in my back.
> 17. I only walk short distances because of my back.
> 18. I sleep less well because of my back.
> 19. Because of my back pain, I get dressed with help from someone else.
> 20. I sit down for most of the day because of my back.
> 21. I avoid heavy jobs around the house because of my back.
> 22. Because of my back pain, I am more irritable and bad tempered with people than usual.
> 23. Because of my back, I go upstairs more slowly than usual.
> 24. I stay in bed most of the time because of my back.
>
> This questionnaire is taken from: Roland MO, Morris RW. A study of the natural history of back pain. Chapter 1: Development of a reliable and sensitive measure of disability in low back pain. Spine 1983; 8: 141–144

Clinical Assessment

Once the subjective questions from the various tools, perhaps including the questionnaires, have been answered, it is time for the clinical expertise of the practitioner to take over.

The range of movement (ROM) of the spine, the willingness to move, any deviation – discrepancy in leg length, for example – the quality of movement and any pain or restriction can all be observed and assessed with a number of clinical tests. Simply observing the ways in which the patient interacts and moves whilst in the treatment room can also be valuable. It may also be good practice, if appropriate and indicated, to assess any neurological deficit, via a 'slump test' (see below).

> ### SLUMP TEST
>
> On occasion, nerves can become more alert and sensitive to the stress placed upon them, for example, in the presence of inflammation or injury. If this is the case then normal movement can cause pain, numbness, tingling or other signs of nerve distress. This is called adverse neural tension, and may cause injury as the body contracts the muscles around the nerves in order to protect them.
>
> The 'slump test' is used to assess adverse neural tension in patients with low-back and hamstring injuries and involves tensioning the neural tissues without additional hamstring stretch. This is achieved by flexing the cervical and thoracic spine during hamstring stretch along the posterior chain. The test may also be used to detect lumbar disc herniation. With the flexed lumbar spine and hip completed simultaneously with the extended leg extension position, the sciatic nerve and its respective nerve roots are put under tension and will indicate the potential diagnosis of a disc herniation. The slump knee bend test and the prone knee bend test both assesses the glide of the femoral nerve anteriorly and have been used to help indicate radicular pain or pain originating as a result of irritation to the spinal structures and may indicate irritation of the nerve roots at L2–L3 due to the innervation of the femoral nerve.
>
> These tests will provide the practitioner with an objective evaluation in the patient's possible level of neural irritation if present.

MUSCULOSKELETAL DISORDERS: THE FINANCIAL COST AND POSSIBLE SOLUTIONS

The neural slump test.

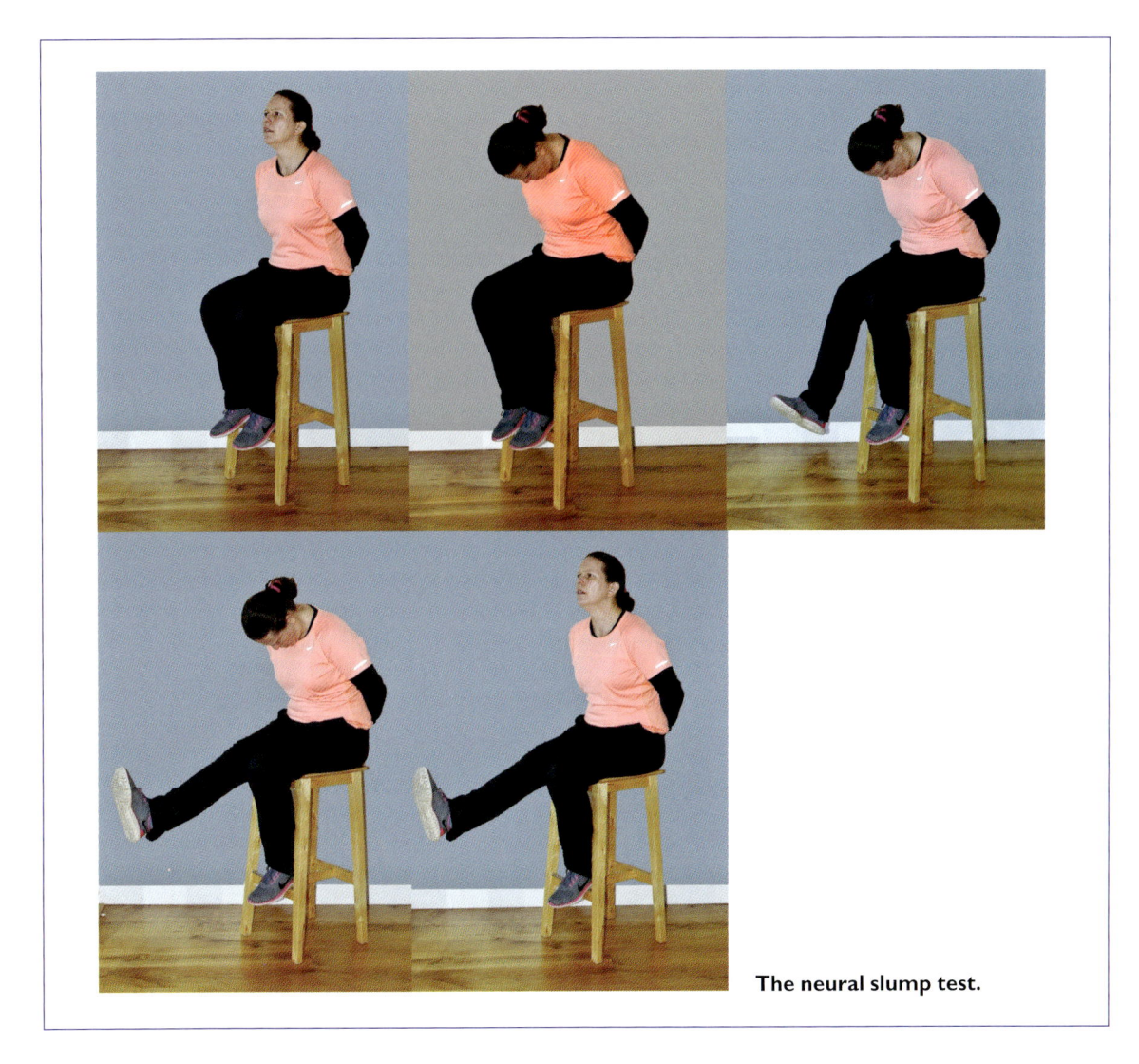

The clinical assessment may also include muscle strength tests. For example, resisted isometrics in flexion, extension, side flexion and rotation can all be manually assessed. Core stability and functional strength tests may also be completed if pain allows.

In the 1950s the Kraus-Webber tests were established and introduced to school-age children in the USA and Europe. The tests involve a series of exercises that measure the strength and flexibility of the back, abdominal, psoas and hamstring muscles. The six positions of assessment are as follows:

- **Kraus Weber Test No. 1.** With the feet held on the ground by the examiner, the subject lies flat on the back with the hands behind the neck. Perform one sit-up.
- **Kraus Weber Test No. 2.** The subject is in the same position except that the knees are bent, with the ankles close to the buttocks. Perform one sit-up.
- **Kraus Weber Test No. 3.** The subject lies flat on the back with the hands behind the neck. The legs are straight and are lifted 10 inches off the floor. Hold this position for 10 seconds.

- **Kraus Weber Test No. 4.** The subject lies on the stomach with a pillow under their lower abdomen and groin. The examiner holds the feet down. Lift head, shoulders, and chest off the floor and hold for 10 seconds.
- **Kraus Weber Test No. 5.** The subject's position is the same as in number 4, but the examiner holds the chest down. With knees straight, lift legs off floor and hold for 10 seconds.
- **Kraus Weber Test No. 6.** The subject stands erect, barefooted, and with feet together. The examiner holds the knees straight. Bend over slowly and touch the floor with the fingertips. Hold this position for 3 seconds.

All of the above tests are graded on a pass-fail basis. The test is passed overall if the subject holds all the positions for the prescribed duration, but a failure to perform even one of the six exercises leads to an overall fail.

Babalola et al. (2008) wanted to determine the strength and flexibility of the spinal and hamstring muscles among University of Ibadan students and the reliability of the Kraus-Weber exercise test within this cohort. In this study of 200 people, 52 per cent of 18- to 30-year-olds failed the test. They concluded that the Kraus-Weber test is reliable and easy to administer. They also recommended within the paper that individuals with weak abdominal and back muscles – in other words, those who failed the test – should be taken through remedial exercises in order to improve their strength and flexibility. It was also suggested that all individuals without low back pain should make a habit of recreational exercise to help strengthen their low back, abdominals, psoas and hamstring muscles.

What is clear is that everyone is vulnerable to low back pain, especially as the ageing process compromises the body in those three main areas already described – reduction in joint mobility; decrease in muscular strength; and slowing of reaction and movement times. Addressing these areas through strength and conditioning will help prevent any future problems and ensure good health, function and physical activity into later life.

Other clinical assessments may include a simple timed plank hold, or a note of the number of either double-leg or single-leg bridging movements with quality that can be completed. Also useful is the core muscle strength and stability test, in which a number of different movement patterns from a plank position are completed for a prescribed duration. The target of the core muscle strength and stability test includes single-arm raise and single-leg raise with alternate legs and arms, all for a 15-second duration, progressing to both arm and leg raises from the plank position, all completed continuously within the test. Standards and scores are all relative and, once the quality of movement is compromised due to fatigue or poor quality, then the test should be stopped, and the total duration recorded.

The sit-up test completed to time – simply the number of sit-ups that the subject can complete in 30 seconds, 1 minute or 2 minutes, for example – is another measure of abdominal strength, as is the sit-up or curl-up test, keeping pace with a metronome. The National Coaching Foundation Abdominal Curl Conditioning Test, available on CD for testing large groups or individuals, is a tempo test. Once the individual is unable to keep up with the pacer or metronome that sets the tempo, then the test is complete, and the total number of repetitions and total duration can be recorded.

It will not be possible to administer these more dynamic tests on a patient with acute or severe back pain, but they can be used to look at baseline levels of strength with a healthy group or asymptomatic individual before injury and perhaps to identify any weaknesses that may need to be addressed prophylactically to prevent future issues and injury, as suggested by Babalola et al. (2008). According to statistics from the Health and Safety Executive, the workforce in the construction industry loses a significant amount of time to injury. It would surely be prudent to assess such a group for strength and then to put in place a scheme whereby each individual has a basic strengthening and mobility plan to follow. The introduction of a basic core conditioning programme would be an effective prevention tool to help reduce the incidence of workforce musculoskeletal injury. The strength tests are valid, repeatable, reliable and easy to administer to a large group, and this is surely an area where companies can save money in loss of workforce due to injury.

Another test that is important to the practitioner is the Gillet Test, which assesses the mobility limitation in the sacroiliac region. The test is completed in standing by raising the knee to 90 degrees. The practitioner will assess how the sacroiliac joint moves on each side via palpation of the patient's posterior superior iliac spine (PSIS). If movement is restricted, then it implies that the sacroiliac joint is compromised, which may affect function and pain. Corrective exercises may then be prescribed.

Biofeedback can also be used to measure the control of the spinal muscles and is a good provider of feedback to the patient, allowing for effective assessment, re-education and training of the muscles in the lumbar spine. Research by Uddin *et al.* (2013) supports the view that the functional integration of stabilizer biofeedback training directed at the deep abdominals and the lumbar muscles is effective in reducing pain and functional disability in patients with chronic low back pain.

Another screening tool that can assess trunk strength and stability is the Functional Movement Screen (FMS), originally launched in 1995. It is used to identify limitations or asymmetries in seven fundamental movement patterns that have been identified as key functional movement qualities in individuals with no current pain complaint or known musculoskeletal injury. The FMS is to be used for healthy, active people and for healthy and inactive people who want to increase physical activity. For those with pain, the Selective Functional Movement Assessment (SFMA) is more appropriate. This movement-based diagnostic system is designed to clinically assess seven fundamental movement patterns in clients or athletes with known musculoskeletal pain. It provides an efficient method for the systematic identification of the cause of symptoms, not just the source, by logically breaking down dysfunctional patterns and diagnosing their root cause as either a mobility problem or a stability/motor control problem. The screen is designed to be conducted by professional qualified clinicians (chartered physiotherapists, osteopaths, orthopaedic medical practitioners, and so on), to help them assess their patient's musculoskeletal evaluation and assist in further corrective exercises and diagnosis.

The seven selective functional movement assessments are as follows:

1. cervical spine movement assessment;
2. upper extremity movement pattern of the shoulder;
3. multi-segmental flexion assessment;
4. multi-segmental extension assessment;
5. multi-segmental rotation assessment;
6. single-leg-stance assessment;
7. overhead deep squat assessment.

There are sub-assessments on most of the above screens as well, to look at movement through range, which should be completed by a qualified practitioner. Core strength, spinal mobility and stability will be evaluated via this assessment. For more detail, *see* functionalmovement.com.

There are many screening and assessment tools and each practitioner will have their favourites that they use when evaluating a patient. The common factor is that, if there is a deficiency, muscle imbalance, mechanical malalignment, over-use or weakness, then over time this is likely to cause problems and lead to pain and, possibly, to restricted movement. An acute onset may require treatment, but it is also worth considering a more proactive approach. All individuals can become aware of their own back health and informed about the likely occurrence of low back pain as they age, and make a conscious choice to prevent any potential problems.

Introducing regular mobility and strength into the daily routine is a good way of doing this.

A sedentary individual may have normal, pain-free function but may be at risk of progressive age-related weakness, which will in turn place them at risk of the onset of back pain. After many episodes of high torque and exposure through work or sports, or daily living, when wear and tear are already likely, all it takes is one heavy lift, incorrect movement, twisting or turning out of synch to cause the pain and spasm associated with acute back pain and the resultant problems.

According to the National Institute of Neurological Disorders and Stroke (2014), the fact is that 80 per cent of adults at some point in their life will experience low back pain and about 20 per cent of people affected by acute low back pain will then develop chronic low back pain, with persistent symptoms at one year. This is a big problem, but perhaps becoming stronger can make a difference.

CHAPTER 3

CASE STUDIES: THE PRACTICAL APPLICATION OF CORE CONDITIONING, PRESCRIPTION AND EXERCISE SELECTION

It is important to consider all the functional requirements of the individual who needs a conditioning programme to help strengthen their core and associated musculature. A programme may involve a number of what may be termed more 'traditional' core exercises, as well as some functional movement patterns that require good postural control and core activation to perform, but will also condition the lower limbs, for example, and lead to improved overall functional performance.

If a limb is moved away from the body, this activates the transversus abdominis, external oblique, lumbar multifidus, and erector spinae, among others. It makes sense to consider all this when training an individual and helping them prepare for functional movement again, especially after injury. In addition, it is important to brace before completing the movement, to stabilize the spine and get the most out of that movement. I talk about 'optimizing the exercise': in other words, getting the maximum benefit from each exercise by completing it with excellent technique, by bracing, contracting, breathing and understanding where the muscles are working. This is known as 'body awareness'; the better the client's body awareness is, the better their outcome.

The case studies below include six examples of specific injuries or issues that may be experienced in the general or sporting population. They will demonstrate how specific core strengthening can be complemented with functional strengthening and movement patterns, leading to a more positive outcome of reconditioning. Sometimes, the injury will have occurred because of a weak core, weak low back or poor control caused by a lack of conditioning. However, becoming stronger through all of the planes of motion, as body control and function improve, will lead to a better outcome for the individual and a more successful return to pain-free activity.

In order to make progress in core training, it will be necessary to advance from the many options of more controlled, isometric activation type prone or supine exercises to standing, walking, single-leg and loaded exercises. Applied conditioning with appropriate overload is the way to improve strength, a dynamic challenge that should lead to long-term success, with a reduction in pain and an increase in function. It would be short-sighted to imagine that a few sit-ups will do the job satisfactorily. With an awareness of the concept of whole-body movements – how moving an arm or a leg causes the muscles around the spine to be activated, to protect the spine – it is possible to select exercises that depending on the client's requirements, will address core strength and stability. However, this should be done in a functional, more applied way, for long-term gain and physical development.

NEEDS ANALYSIS

In planning a programme, it will be necessary to gain an insight into the client's lifestyle. An understanding of their commitments, access to facilities, injury history, sports completed and time available are all very important factors to consider with any exercise prescription. Knowing what their outcome goals are will also help with planning a specific programme for their requirements. A thorough needs analysis should be completed in order to consider how best to positively affect the individual and to help create a profile for them. This, with any accompanying clinical notes from their practitioner – GP, musculoskeletal specialist, osteopath, chartered physiotherapist, athletic trainer or other professional – will provide an essential insight into their requirements. A multidisciplinary approach will also identify any possible contraindications, which is always valuable, especially in more complicated cases, such as a prolapsed disc. The more information there is available at this stage of planning the exercise prescription, the more likely it is that the needs of the individual will be addressed and a positive outcome will be achieved.

A needs analysis form might look like the following:

Needs Analysis

Client name	
Occupation	
Address	
Email address	
Mobile number	
DOB/age	
Sports/physical activities completed	
Training history	
Injury history *Please include date of injury, surgical dates, investigations/scans, left/right side, etc. Please be as specific as possible.*	
Goals/training targets *e.g. stronger legs, leaner, general fitness improvement, upcoming events and dates*	

CASE STUDIES: THE PRACTICAL APPLICATION OF CORE CONDITIONING

Commitments *e.g. work, family, time constraints, etc.*	
Gym access and facilities	
Referring practitioner (if relevant)	
Any other relevant information	

Please complete the information below as thoroughly as possible and send any associated clinical communication, scans, reports, etc. to complement the detail below. Thank you.
This is what I will base your exercise prescription on, so the more detail, the better.
Your answers will be treated in the strictest confidence.

Once the information has been completed, it will be used as the basis for planning a conditioning programme, targeting any corrective exercises and necessary conditioning for the individual. Each programme will give direction regarding frequency, duration and intensity, to allow the client to make the right choices regarding when they complete their plan and how they should feel during and after it. They must have an understanding of and be accountable for their programme. They will be given the tools and information to be successful and, most importantly, develop their body awareness to ensure that they have a positive outcome from this intervention. This is very important after injury or if someone is in pain.

RATING OF PERCEIVED EXERTION

One of the most important areas in rehabilitation and conditioning is the intensity of the session. This is often missed in exercise prescription and, if the intensity is too low or too high, it can affect a number of factors. For example, if the individual is too sore to complete the next session because of severe DOMS (delayed onset muscle soreness), then adherence can be affected. Some DOMS is acceptable, but not if it is debilitating! Conversely, it may be that the intensity is too low and the sessions will not cause an appropriate overload stimulus to make a positive physiological change. This needs to be communicated to the individual as confidence increases intensity and loading needs to increase. I use the term 'threshold' with the client. Ideally, they should be just below their personal threshold, so that they work hard and improve, but not beyond their threshold, which would cause an increased injury risk or severe DOMS.

The individual should be guided on intensity using the Borg Rating of Perceived Exertion Scale (see below).

Rating of Perceived Exertion: RPE Scale

0	Rest
1	Very very easy
2	Easy
3	Moderate
4	Somewhat hard
5	Hard
6	
7	Very hard
8	
9	
10	Maximal

Borg, G. (1998) *Borg's perceived exertion and pain scales. Human Kinetics.*

The RPE Scale gives a quantitative identification of the feeling of fatigue. It indicates a subjective sensation of effort. These feelings of fatigue are very highly correlated with the intensity of exercise.

Borg gives the following instructions (*Borg's Perceived Exertion and Pain Scales*, 1998):

> Each day estimate how hard you feel your exercise workload is.
>
> This feeling should reflect your total amount of exertion and fatigue, combining all sensations and inner feelings of physical stress, effort and fatigue. Focus on the entire body. Try not to underestimate or overestimate your feeling or exertion. Be as accurate as you can.

I use the Borg 0–10 scale for both a measure of exercise intensity as well as for a pain scale – it is important for clients who have pain to understand how they feel: 0 = no pain and 10 = maximal pain. As the client becomes familiar with the tool, using it for both feelings of exertion/intensity as well as pain will hopefully lead to consistency of reporting and feedback from the individual. This is very important when dealing with clients who have frequent pain and are symptomatic.

In view of the fact that pain can lead to depression and depression can lead to pain, it is important to track how an individual is coping with their programme. If something is recorded as significantly higher than I was planning it to be, it may alert me to look at things in a little more detail for the client. Programmes need to be fluid and adaptable as things change, and trust is very important in the relationship between the client and the strength and conditioning coach. The client needs to be able to trust that what the coach has prescribed will not cause any further pain or problems. That relationship cannot be underestimated in regard to outcome. Reassurance, body awareness and an empathy with the individual are all important skills for the S&C coach.

CASE STUDIES: REAL LIFE APPLICATION

The following are a number of case studies that involve issues or injury to the core area and associated musculature. Sometimes, the injury may not even be seemingly associated to a core strength deficiency or imbalance, yet, if the core and posterior chain are strengthened, pain caused by a lack of core conditioning can be reduced. This ability to look at the whole picture with a client is essential.

I see a significant number of people who have already visited three or four different practitioners to solve a problem, pain or injury, who discover that simply becoming stronger in the right way allows them to wave goodbye to their pain. It is about being fit for purpose, robust and strong, and a good S&C coach will give all clients an appropriate applied conditioning programme. Using case studies to present my conditioning and reconditioning/rehabilitation ideas and philosophy will hopefully allow for an applied sharing of knowledge. The aim is to help both individuals who are living with pain and the practitioners who are employed or engaged in a return-to-action package for clients or patients. These real-life examples have made a difference to the quality of life and function for the individuals involved. All required an improvement in their body awareness, and the application of processes to enable the body to become stronger. Once function improved and pain subsided, they were able to progress on to more demanding exercises that ultimately enabled a return to sport or pain-free daily life.

My philosophy is a positive one. I believe that, by becoming stronger and ensuring an appropriate balance between mobility and strength, it is possible to re-educate the body to move well, retrain and regain its function, hopefully allowing for a return to pain-free living. Pain can be debilitating, not only for the individual concerned but also for their family. It can have a huge psychological effect

CASE STUDIES: THE PRACTICAL APPLICATION OF CORE CONDITIONING

on wellbeing and mental health and this should be considered when working with individuals who have potential life-affecting injury and associated pain. Having empathy and understanding for each client is important, as they need to believe in you and your programme. This is especially true when someone is in pain. Gaining a client's trust, helping them to believe that what you prescribe will help them, even in the early stages when pain may still be present, is essential. Trust, adherence and motivation are all part of the on-going working relationship between client and practitioner.

As an S&C specialist I usually have clients referred to me when they are just out of an acute injury phase, or post-surgery. They may have seen a physiotherapist or sports medicine specialist, who has recommended some specific strength and conditioning so that they may make further progress. They can function and move but not to the level that they desire. Sometimes, they just want to improve and get over that final hurdle to full function. Others may be more ambitious, with a desire to return to full-contact or high-performance sport.

Changes in the body may only be achieved through being proactive, motivated, driven and accountable. Even the best rehabilitation programme will not work unless it is actioned. If the client does action it, it is likely to make a difference.

I work with busy, professional people, who do not particularly have time in their life for conditioning. However, they are also people who need to make a positive change to their physical wellbeing and function, to prevent it having a negative effect on their quality of life. A proper understanding of a client and their time limitations may lead an S&C coach to prescribe, for example, 3 x 20-minute session chunks instead of a 60-minute session. This may mean the difference between a client completing the plan and not doing so! Communication is key. An open, honest relationship will ensure trust and best outcome.

All the case studies will involve some core, posterior chain, lumbar spine, associated issue or injury, and a conditioning plan is provided for each example. They include injury rehabilitation cases associated with poor core strength and stability. Many people put up with pain or accept their own personal best function. Striving to be better by becoming stronger is a really positive thing and will hopefully lead to a fit and healthy, pain-free life.

The focus for most of the case studies below is high-volume exercises, to encourage body awareness and endurance/adaptation and neural recruitment. Reduced repetitions and increased load represent a natural progression for most clients, but most exercises are based around muscular endurance and hypertrophy sets and repetitions or duration, and then progressed to more strength-based loading, depending on the client's requirements, age and goals. Many of these clients have detrained or have no training background, so the prescribed sets, repetitions and loading need to reflect this. I find with rehabilitation that often repetition of a movement pattern and resultant muscle memory is very useful to ensure a good foundation and understanding early in the programme, especially if the individual has low training exposure or history. Recommendations in loading, sets and repetition selection should be applied in context to the individual and should be contingent upon an individual's target goals, physical capacity and training status.

The case studies have been selected to provide guidance when prescribing exercises to an individual, but it is important to recognize that everyone is different. What works for one client may or may not work well for another. These case studies should however help with optimizing a core and associated strength programme, with exercise selections and progressions that can be used and understood in an applied setting.

These are actual case studies from people I have managed. They have all been asked to raise any concern over their inclusion here and their identity has been removed for confidentiality.

CASE STUDIES: THE PRACTICAL APPLICATION OF CORE CONDITIONING

CASE STUDY 1

Assessment

Diagnosis: prolapsed/herniated disc (also known as a slipped disc)

Definition: in the case of a prolapsed or herniated disc (also known as a slipped disc), one of the discs of cartilage in the spine is damaged and pressing on the nerves. A slipped disc occurs when the circle of connective tissue surrounding the disc breaks down, allowing the soft, inner gel-like part of the disc to bulge out. The damaged disc can put pressure on the whole spinal cord or on a single nerve root, where a nerve leaves the spinal cord. This means a slipped disc can cause pain in the area of the protruding disc and also in the area of the body controlled by the nerve on which the disc is pressing (https://www.nhs.uk/conditions/slipped-disc).

Needs Analysis

Client name	Client # 1
Occupation	Student.
DOB/age	23 years old.
Sports/physical activities completed	Recreational only. Rugby from age 11–16, skiing from a young age to present, racquet sports.
Training history	Gym: primarily free weights, strength focused. 16 years old to present day. Not much cardio completed.
Injury history *Please include date of injury, surgical dates, investigations/scans, left/right side, etc. Please be as specific as possible.*	Slipped disc between L5 and S1 vertebrae, fused to nerve of right leg, significantly reduced flexibility and mobility. History of hamstring tear in right leg. Steroid injection into lumbar region 6 months ago. No change in symptoms.
Goals/training targets *e.g. stronger legs, leaner, general fitness improvement, upcoming events and dates*	Increase flexibility and mobility. Regain strength.
Commitments *e.g. work, family, time constraints, etc.*	At university: studies.
Gym access and facilities	Home gym and gym access at university. Vibration platform and weights available at home.
Referring practitioner (if relevant)	Self-referral.
Any other relevant information	Nil.

CASE STUDIES: THE PRACTICAL APPLICATION OF CORE CONDITIONING

Current presentation:
Sore whilst sitting and in bed. Restriction when playing sport. Long-term pain and restricted movement. Very frustrated.

Exercise prescription:
Prescribed session to be completed 3–4 x each week. Emphasis on quality of movement and attention to detail with prescribed movement patterns.

Other things to consider:
Targets:
- Increase flexibility and mobility.
- Strength improvement.
- Desire to play recreational sport including tag rugby and racquet sports.

Challenges/concerns:
History is worrisome in a 23-year-old. Already had a steroid injection into lumbar area to help try to relieve symptoms to no avail. Excellent focus and adherence to the programme. The client wants to improve his quality of life.

Strength and Conditioning Plan

Checklist:
- Improve mobility via spinal mobility plan and dynamic mobility/myofascial release/PNF/Vibration training to help increase lower limb ROM.
- Improve core strength and activation to off-load the spine.
- Improve hamstring range of movement via progressive strength loading.
- Improve general lower limb strength via functional exercises.
- Do spinal mobility exercises 2 x daily (see table).
- Do range of movement exercises 3 to 4 x each week (see table).

Frequency:
- Mobility to be completed 2 x daily (morning and evening).

Spinal Mobility

Exercise	Sets	Reps	Comments
Lumbar rolls	2	10 x L and R	Work through a full ROM.
Lumbar rotations	2	10 x L and R	
Cat stretch and downward dog	2	3 blocks of 3 = 1 set	
Back extension	2	10	
Seated slumps	2	8 x L and R	Very restricted movement: unable to extend fully.

Range of Movement Exercises

Exercise	Sets/reps/rest	Comments
Vibration platform	3 x 30 seconds. Work alternate leg	Hamstring stretch position. Ensure hips/pelvis are square and not tilted or uneven.
Myofascial release	2 x 45 seconds on quads, hamstrings, ITB, glutes and calves	Foam roller or tennis ball/peanut used.
Dynamic/static stretches: static calf stretches and dynamic hamstring stretches	Calf static stretches: 3 x 30 seconds L and R Sweep the floor/chase the chickens L and R alternate sides x 2 x 10	Good position in dynamic hamstrings. Posture: don't cheat and move into poor movement patterns as lower limb ROM is a challenge.

49

CASE STUDIES: THE PRACTICAL APPLICATION OF CORE CONDITIONING

- Core strength programme to be completed 3–4 x each week.
- Range of movement exercises to be completed 3–4 x each week.
- Supplementary exercises to be completed 2–3 x each week.

Session duration:
Mobility = 10 minutes
Core strength = 30–40 minutes
Range of movement exercises = 5–10 minutes
Supplementary exercises = 15–20 minutes

Intensity:
Borg Rating of Perceived Exertion (RPE) = 5–6–7 (hard–very hard)
Pain scale: <2–3 (easy–moderate) (Borg RPE used for pain scale)

Note to client:

- All exercises should be completed with absolute attention to detail and with excellent technique.
- If the quality of movement is compromised because of fatigue or pain, rest and then go again.
- Improve body awareness and know where you should feel the muscles work.
- Consider your breathing technique: belly breathe out and brace: feel the muscles contract in your core and blow out when instructed, as if you are blowing a ping pong ball away.

Core Strengthening Plan

- Select 4–6 exercises in each session.
- Vary the choice for each session and complete with excellent control.

- Complete these exercises 3–4 times each week in addition to your prescribed S&C programme.

THE CLAM
3 sets left and right to fatigue (feel the burn!)

- Perform this exercise without a band to begin with (unlike in the image).
- Side lie on the floor and bend your knees together.
- Relax your upper body and activate your core (brace and pull).
- Start with the hips and shoulders square then externally rotate the hip (lift it off the other knee).
- Try to keep the rest of the body stationary as the hip rotates.
- Return to the start position and repeat for the prescribed number of sets and repetitions in a slow and controlled manner.

LONG LEVER: BAND HIP ABDUCTION
- 3 x left and right side to fatigue.
- Rest = 5 seconds then repeat.
- Switch legs after all 3 sets.

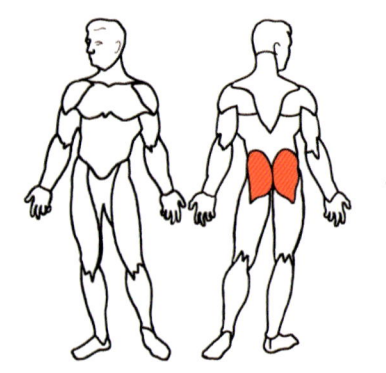

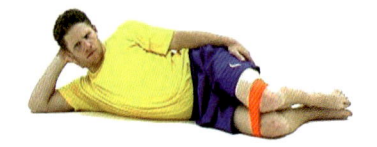

The clam.

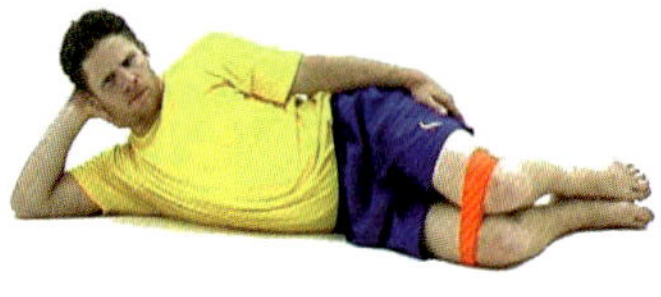

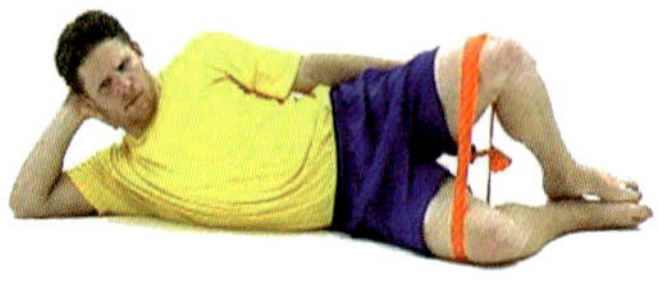

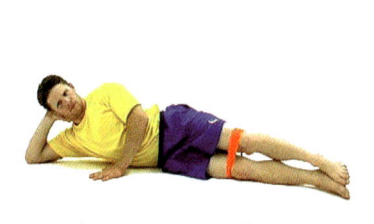

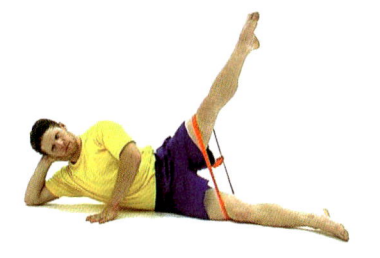

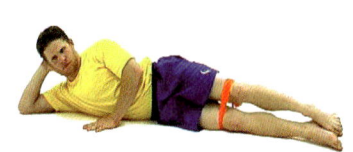

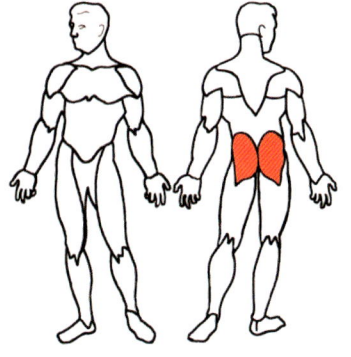

CASE STUDIES: THE PRACTICAL APPLICATION OF CORE CONDITIONING

Long lever: band hip abduction.

FRONT PLANK

20–30 second holds x 4–5 repetitions.
5 seconds rest in between sets.

- Start with the forearms flat on the floor with the palms facing down.
- Extend the hips and knees to press up to a front support position while keeping the torso rigid.
- Ensure that your back is in a strong position with your bottom slightly raised.
- Brace this position and try to contract the glutes.
- Hold the position for 20–30 seconds and complete 4–5 repetitions with 5 seconds rest in between sets.
- Use your breathing: big 'belly breath' and brace.

Caution: keep the neck in line with the spine and do not allow the spine to sag or drop.

DOUBLE-LEG/SINGLE-LEG BRIDGING

Raise up with two legs, then switch to single leg, then return to floor with control. Complete as prescribed below:

3 x 10 repetitions left and right, hold each raise/rep for 3–4 seconds. Belly breathe and brace.

- Start with the feet approximately shoulder width apart with the head and shoulders in contact with the ground.
- Lift the hips off the ground until the thighs are in line with the torso.
- Then lift one leg up and straight out, in line with your body.

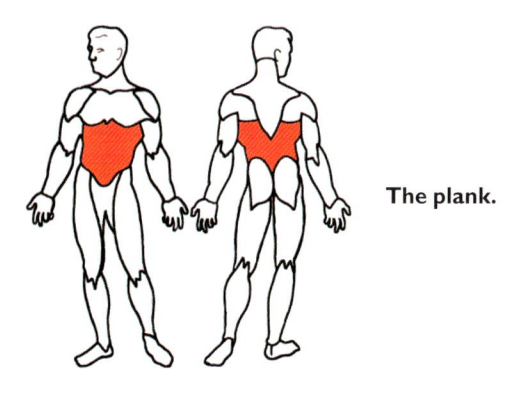

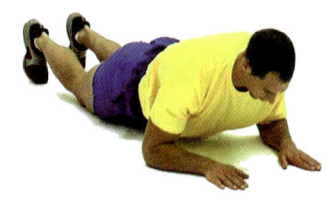

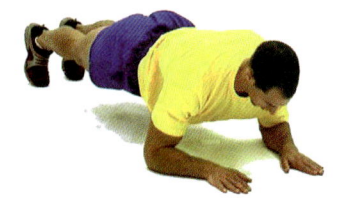

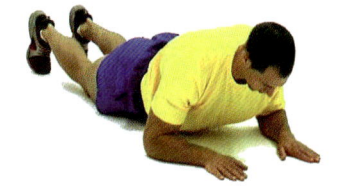

The plank.

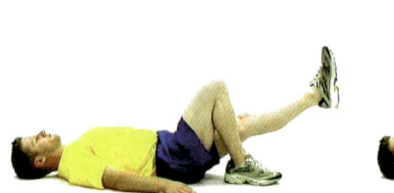

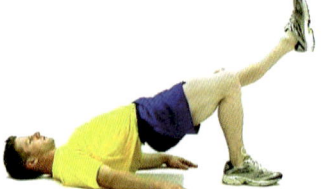

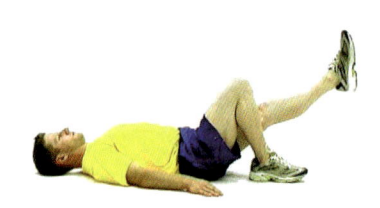

CASE STUDIES: THE PRACTICAL APPLICATION OF CORE CONDITIONING

- Hold for 3–4 seconds, and then control the movement of your bottom back to the start position.
- Continue with the same leg for the prescribed number of repetitions.
- Switch legs after the repetitions have been completed.
- Breathe throughout the exercise and brace when raised.

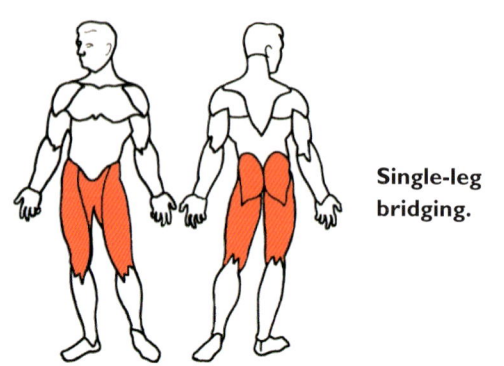

SUPINE SWISS BALL BRIDGING WITH HIP FLEXION

3 x 30 second holds.

Progressing to 3 x 10 repetitions left and right, hold each raise/rep for 3–4 seconds. Belly breathe and brace as you lift.

- Start with the head and shoulders on the stability ball with the knees in line with the hips and the feet under the knees.
- Maintain the bridging position for the prescribed duration.
- Progression: lift one foot off the ground then place it back on to the ground.
- Hold for 2–3 seconds.
- Repeat the movements with alternate legs continuously with excellent control.
- Place the hands across the chest, out wide or above the head while maintaining the same body position, to vary and progress the exercise.

Single-leg bridging.

Caution: maintain a neutral spine and level pelvic position and do not allow the lower back to extend excessively.

KNEELING ARM-LEG RAISE

3 x 10 repetitions left and right (20 total alternate reps).

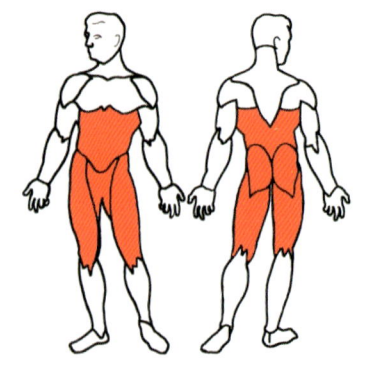

Supine Swiss ball bridging with hip flexion.

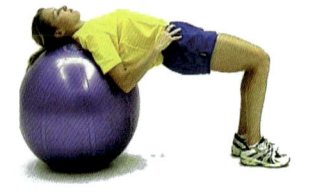

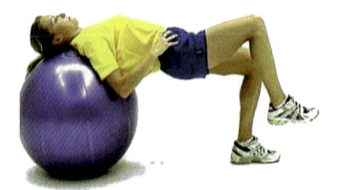

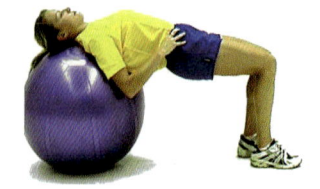

CASE STUDIES: THE PRACTICAL APPLICATION OF CORE CONDITIONING

Kneeling arm-leg raise.

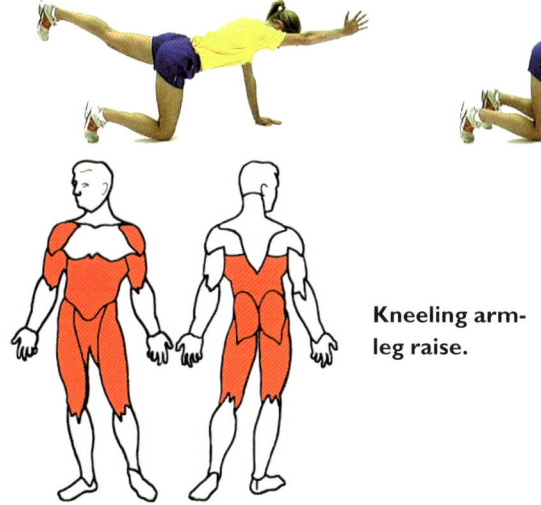

Place a tennis ball in the small of your back if possible to ensure no sway and for feedback.

- Start with the hands under the shoulders, the knees under the hips and neutral curves of the spine.
- Brace and breathe as you extend a leg/arm, breathe in on return phase, maintaining the brace.
- Extend the hip and knee and extend the opposite shoulder.
- Hold for 3 seconds then return back to the four-point kneeling position with excellent control and no sway.
- Repeat the movements with both limbs in an alternating fashion for the prescribed number of sets and repetitions.

Caution: do not allow the spine to round or sag, especially as you get fatigued.

ALTERNATING HIP FLEXION/EXTENSION
3 x 10 left and right alternating.
5 seconds rest in between each set.

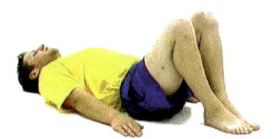

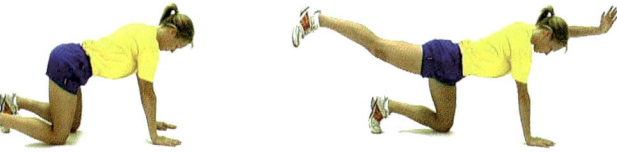

Extend legs further and add arms overhead as a progression.

- Start with the hips and knees flexed to 90 degrees on the floor.
- Contrary to the image, keep your head and neck on the floor throughout the exercise.
- Breathe out and brace during the extension phase (straight leg) for each leg, breathe in on the flexion (bent leg) phase.
- Flex and extend the legs for the prescribed number of repetitions with excellent control.
- The speed of the movement should be slow and controlled, approximately 2–3 seconds for each leg extension movement out and 2–3 seconds for the return movement. Tempo: 3-1-3.

Caution: do not forcefully flex the neck during the exercise; keep your head on the floor throughout the exercise (unlike the image); make sure your back stays in contact with the floor and does not arch upwards during the exercises. If it does, your leg is extending too far, so you need to extend slightly less.

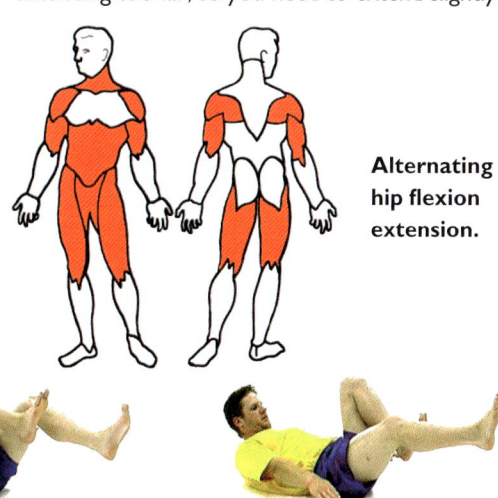

Alternating hip flexion extension.

53

CASE STUDIES: THE PRACTICAL APPLICATION OF CORE CONDITIONING

Additional/Supplementary Conditioning Exercises

Exercise	Sets x reps and rest	Rationale	Comments
Glute band activation: crab walks	3 x L and R to fatigue	Glute conditioning/overload/activation.	Slow and controlled, dedicated movement.
Swiss ball curls	3 x 6–8 double leg; progress to single leg control 15 seconds rest	Good lumbar spine, glute and hamstring activation and strength/control.	Maintain bridge position.
Stability ball single leg squat	3 x 8 L and R Work alternate leg	Great for lower limb control: target = 90 degrees flexion. Stability in the pelvis, glutes, quads/hamstrings also good proprioceptive control.	Very hard to complete: a certain imbalance and requirement to improve single leg control.
Single leg step-up: front and lateral	3 x 12 L and R Work alternate leg	Lower limb functional movement: Co-contraction of lower limbs to allow smooth movement. Good muscular endurance/capacity.	Progress load over coming weeks.
Romanian dead lift	4 x 8 30 seconds rest	Strength loading with RDL used to help improve functional range of movement (ROM) with client as this was a limiting factor in his hamstrings.	Positive progress made with RDL. Good technique and body awareness.
Split squats	3 x 12 L and R Work alternate leg (no rest)	Inclusion was to develop lower limb endurance capacity after detraining/lack of activity.	Client found this hard, but it was a finisher and progression in load and capacity was good over the weeks.

Progressions

Exercises were progressed as follows:

1. Increased load progression: worked to a repetition maximum. The client began with body weight to begin with then via external load (dumbbell/barbell). He progressed well.
2. Decreased stability: exercises completed on BOSU/Swiss ball, ball balanced on back, for example to increase challenge and body feedback/awareness.

Progressions of exercise selection:

- The clam and long lever hip abduction progressed to using the mini band and also pulsing to add intensity and overload.
- Front plank progressed to leg lift, arm lift and to plank rotation.
- Double-leg bridging progressed to single-leg bridging, which then progressed to bridging on a Swiss ball, again double-leg progressing to single-leg.

CASE STUDIES: THE PRACTICAL APPLICATION OF CORE CONDITIONING

- Supine Swiss ball bridging progressed to better-quality hip flexion/leg lift holds, in addition to moving arms overhead with progressive load: dumbbells and weight plate. Progressed to figure eight with load whilst maintaining excellent position and leg lift.
- Kneeling arm-leg raise progressed with load via dumbbells as well as a ball placed on lower back to ensure no sway/rotation.
- Medicine ball wood chop whole-body exercises introduced: more dynamic movement pattern.
- Racquet sport movement patterns introduced: rotation activities and lunge patterns on BOSU.
- Other core exercises were added in, for example seated oblique rotation with a medicine ball.

Outcome

- I saw the client on average once and sometimes twice a week for 5 months.
- At no point during any of the exercises did he experience back pain.
- His adherence to the programme was outstanding.
- His body awareness and 'coachability' were excellent.
- His level of function improved significantly: getting in and out of bed and sleeping became pain-free. Normal daily activities became pain-free and fluid.
- He felt confident for a return to sport, which is an excellent outcome.
- His range of movement through his hamstrings became significantly improved. Before the programme he felt like his hamstrings would 'snap' if he had to bend down or run; this sensation has gone away.
- Clinically this client is asymptomatic and has improved his level of function significantly. His levels of strength and control have improved greatly and he has given himself a great opportunity for good back health over the years to come.

CASE STUDY 2

Assessment

Diagnosis: Pars defect: spondylolisthesis

Definition:
Pars defect: spondylolisthesis is where a bone in the spine (vertebrae) slips out of position, either forwards or backwards. It is most common in the lower back (lumbar spine), but it can also occur in the mid to upper back (thoracic spine) or the neck (cervical spine). There are five main types of spondylolisthesis, each with a different cause. Spondylolisthesis can be caused by the following:

- A birth defect in part of the vertebra.
- Repetitive trauma to the spine: this results in a defect developing in the vertebra, which can cause it to slip; this is known as isthmic spondylolisthesis and is more common in athletes such as gymnasts and weightlifters.
- The joints of the vertebrae becoming worn and arthritic: this is known as degenerative spondylolisthesis and is more common in older people.
- A sudden injury or trauma to the spine: such as a fracture, which can result in the vertebra slipping forward (traumatic spondylolisthesis).
- A bone abnormality: this could be caused by a tumour, for example pathologic spondylolisthesis (https://www.nhs.uk/conditions/spondylolisthesis).

Current presentation:
Low back pain. Pain scale = 4. Sore in daily activities: sitting and walking/standing on occasion. Physiotherapy has helped.

Exercise prescription:
Prescribed session to be completed 3 x each week.
Core strength work: 3–4 x each week.
Emphasis on quality of movement and attention to detail with prescribed movement patterns.

CASE STUDIES: THE PRACTICAL APPLICATION OF CORE CONDITIONING

Needs Analysis

Client name	Client # 2
Occupation	Student
DOB/Age	17 years
Sports/physical activities completed	A keen sportsman and regularly plays football, rugby and Gaelic football.
Training history	Regular sports at school and for clubs. 3–4 x per week.
Injury history *Please include date of injury, surgical dates, investigations/scans, left/right side, etc. Please be as specific as possible.*	MRI scan confirmed stress response and fracture of the right L5 pars interarticularis. Pain onset approximately 5 months ago. MRI thereafter. Has been completing physiotherapy for past 4 months and is now ready to progress loading and function.
Goals/training targets *e.g. stronger legs, leaner, general fitness improvement,* *upcoming events and dates*	Recover fully from fracture. Regain pain-free function. Return to full contact sport. Become stronger.
Commitments *e.g. work, family, time constraints, etc.*	GCSE exams
Gym access and facilities	Member of a gym
Referring practitioner (if relevant)	Local physiotherapist
Any other relevant information	Nil

Static/isometric strength progressing to more dynamic strength progressions for posterior chain and core.

Other things to consider:
Targets:

- Improve confidence for day-to-day movements.
- Strength and muscle activation improvement.
- Age considerations: adolescence and growth to consider and respect. Add in static stretches: quadriceps and calves specifically for growth plates.

Challenges/concerns:
Sessions with chartered physiotherapist have created good general baseline of strength and control. My job is to move the client on to a more functional strength base ensuring that this increase in load and demand does not cause any problems or issues. Create confidence.

Strength and Conditioning Plan

Checklist:

- Ensure excellent understanding of exercises and positions.

CASE STUDIES: THE PRACTICAL APPLICATION OF CORE CONDITIONING

- Continue to improve body awareness and how something should 'feel' when completed.
- Recognize other stressors: studying for GCSEs, peers, etc.

Frequency:
Core strength programme to be completed 3–4 × each week.
Supplementary exercises to be completed 3 × each week.

Session duration:
Core strength = 30 minutes
Supplementary exercises = 30 minutes

Intensity:
Borg Rating of Perceived Exertion (RPE) = 4–5 (moderate–hard)
Target pain scale: <2–3 (easy–moderate) (Borg RPE used for pain scale)

Note to client:

- All exercises should be completed with absolute attention to detail and with excellent technique.
- 'Brace' position through your core, position of strength and belly breath to activate your muscles.
- If the quality of movement is compromised or things become sloppy because of fatigue, rest and then go again.
- Work on your body awareness and know where you should feel the muscles work.

Core Strengthening Plan

- Complete the exercises below 3–4 times each week in addition to your prescribed additional reconditioning programme.
- Select 6–7 out of the 10 options to complete in each session. Make sure you vary the selection.

WARM-UP: GLUTE BAND ACTIVATION
Complete 3 sets of left and right sidewalks or diagonal walks to fatigue.

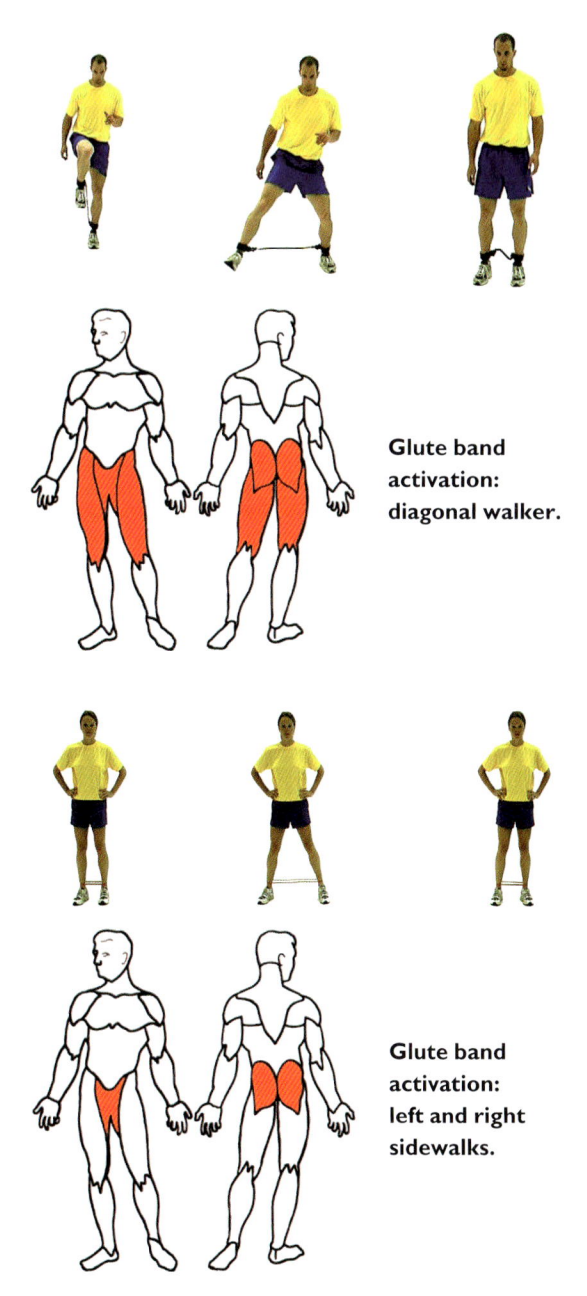

Glute band activation: diagonal walker.

Glute band activation: left and right sidewalks.

- Secure the band around the feet and walk sideways or diagonally while keeping the legs straight.
- Place the hands forward for balance if need be.
- Increase the length of the steps or decrease the contact time with the ground to modify the exercise.

CASE STUDIES: THE PRACTICAL APPLICATION OF CORE CONDITIONING

Caution: ensure that the band is secure and strong enough to withstand the tension developed during this exercise.

SINGLE LEG BRIDGING

3 x 8 left and right side.
Rest = alternate leg.

- Start with the feet approximately shoulder width apart with the head and shoulders in contact with the ground.
- Lift the hips off the ground until the thighs are in line with the torso.
- Then lift one leg up and straight out, in line with your body.
- Hold for 2–3 seconds, and then control the movements back to the start position.

SWISS BALL CURLS

3 sets of 6–8 repetitions.
20 seconds rest in between each set.

- Position the feet securely on the stability ball with the hands on the floor.
- Lift the hips off the floor until the legs are in line with the torso then flex the legs to bring the ball towards the hips with one leg.
- Return back to the start position with one leg.
- Vary the position of the hands on the floor to assist with balance and place the hands across the chest to progress the difficulty of the exercise.
- Complete the prescribed number of sets and reps.

Caution: do not raise the body too high off the floor.

KNEELING ARM-LEG RAISE

3 x 10 repetitions left and right (20 total alternate reps).

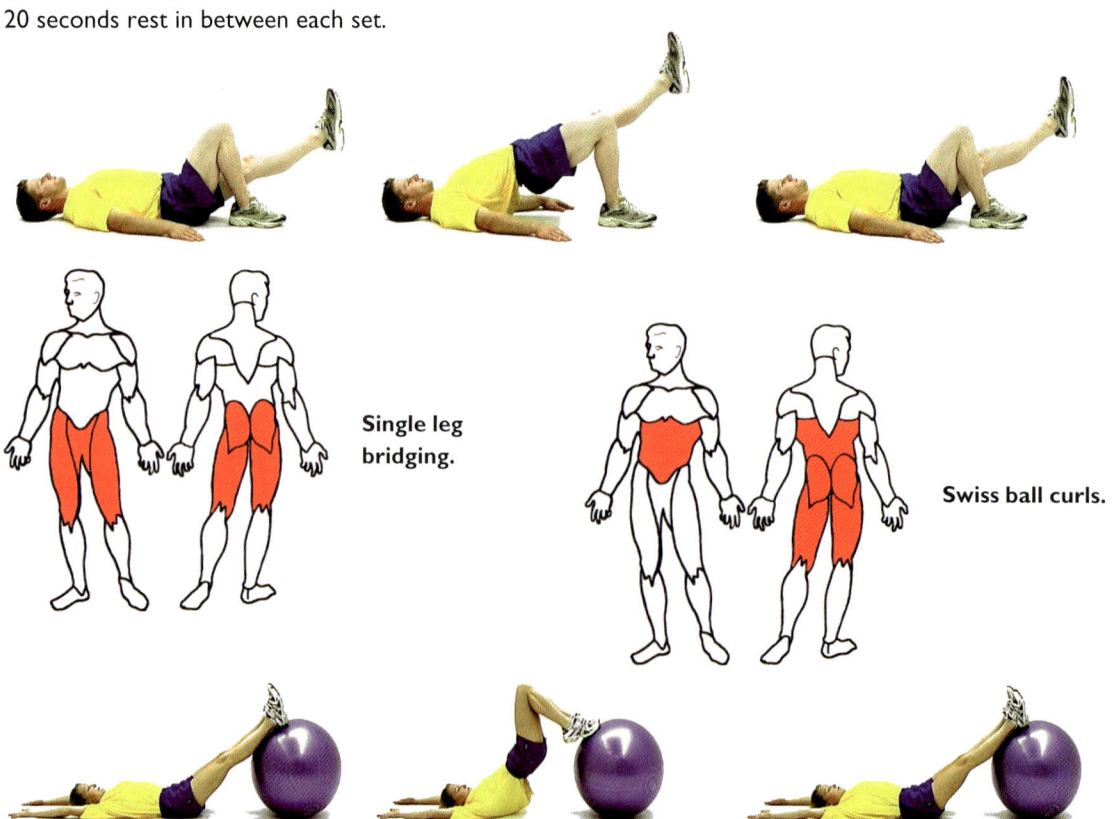

Single leg bridging.

Swiss ball curls.

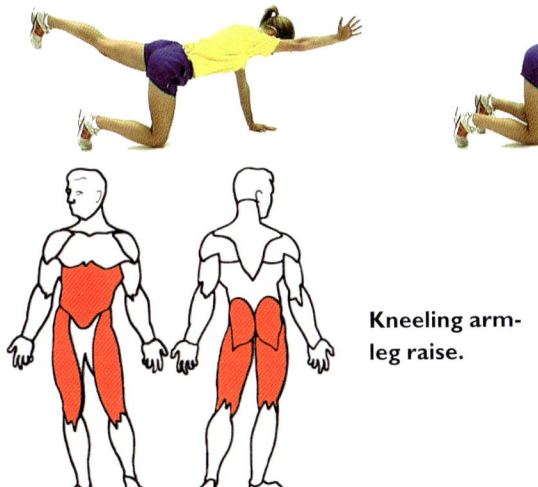

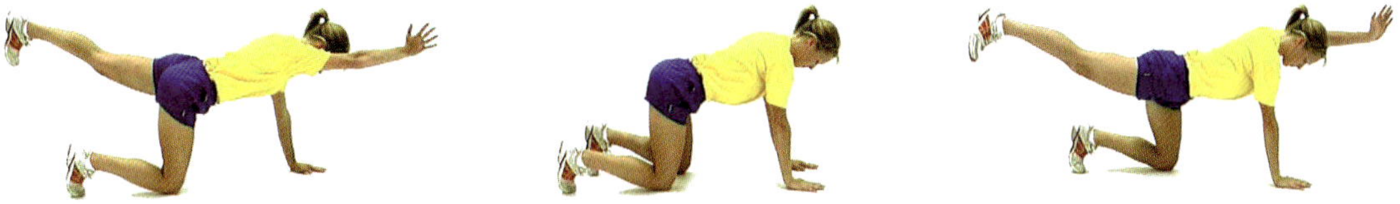

CASE STUDIES: THE PRACTICAL APPLICATION OF CORE CONDITIONING

Kneeling arm-leg raise.

Place a tennis ball in the small of your back if possible to ensure no sway and for feedback.

- Start with the hands under the shoulders, the knees under the hips and neutral curves of the spine.
- Extend the hip and knee and extend the opposite shoulder.
- Hold for 3 seconds then return back to the four-point kneeling position with excellent control and no sway.
- Repeat the movements with both limbs in an alternating fashion for the prescribed number of sets and repetitions.

Caution: do not allow the spine to round or sag, especially as you get fatigued.

PRONE HIP EXTENSION 1
3 x 8–10 repetitions left and right side.
30 seconds rest in between: maintain excellent technique and rest if technique is compromised.

- Lie flat on the stomach with the chin resting on the back of the hands.
- Contract the buttock muscle first and then raise the leg off the ground, keeping the leg straight.
- Reverse the actions to return the leg to the ground.
- Repeat the subsequent repetitions immediately with muscles contracted.

Caution: keep the pelvis square as the leg is raised; avoid rotating the pelvis and do not hyper-extend the spine.

PRONE HIP EXTENSION 2
3 x 8–10 repetitions.
30 seconds rest in between: maintain excellent technique and rest if technique is compromised.

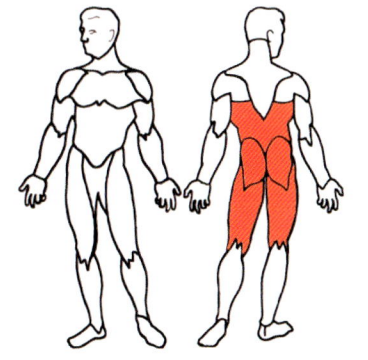

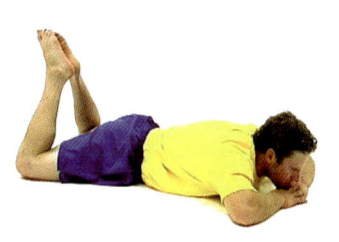

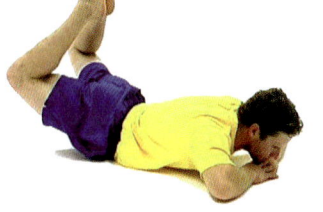

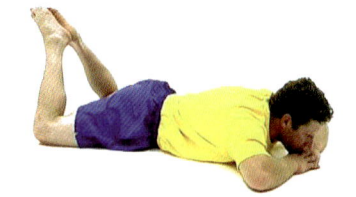

Prone hip extension 1.

CASE STUDIES: THE PRACTICAL APPLICATION OF CORE CONDITIONING

Prone hip extension 2.

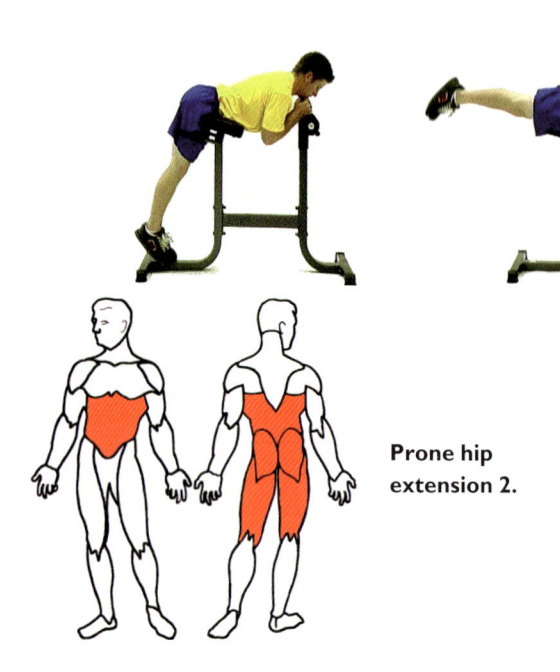

- Hold firmly on to the bench to keep the upper body stable and the neck in line with the spine.
- Raise both legs in unison until the legs are in line with or slightly higher than the position of the spine.
- Reverse the movement to lower the legs back to the start position.
- The range of movement may depend on the requirements of the exercise.
- Complete with excellent control and use your breathing to help.

CRAWLER: FORWARD PRONE WALK

Complete with excellent technique. Rest when the quality of movement goes.
Complete 4 repetitions x 5 metre crawls forwards and backwards = 1 set.
Complete 3–4 sets.
30 seconds rest in between each set.

- Start with the hands under the shoulders and the knees under the hips.
- Keep the shoulder blades flat against the ribs.
- Maintaining neutral curves in the spine, walk forward by pressing off the same hand and foot.

Caution: do not round the shoulders or flex the spine.

BAND HIP EXTENSION AND BAND FLEXION COMPLETED TOGETHER

Complete together with excellent technique. Swing through your hips; *do not* hinge through your back.

- Secure the band or tubing around the lower leg and hold on to something for additional balance if necessary.
- Keep the leg straight and extend the hip as far as comfortable while keeping the shoulders above the hips.

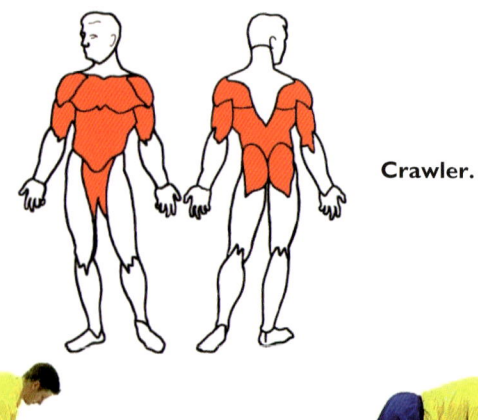

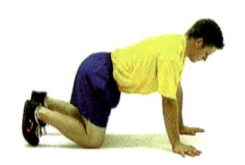

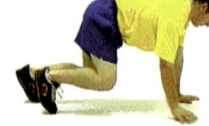

Crawler.

60

CASE STUDIES: THE PRACTICAL APPLICATION OF CORE CONDITIONING

Band hip extension.

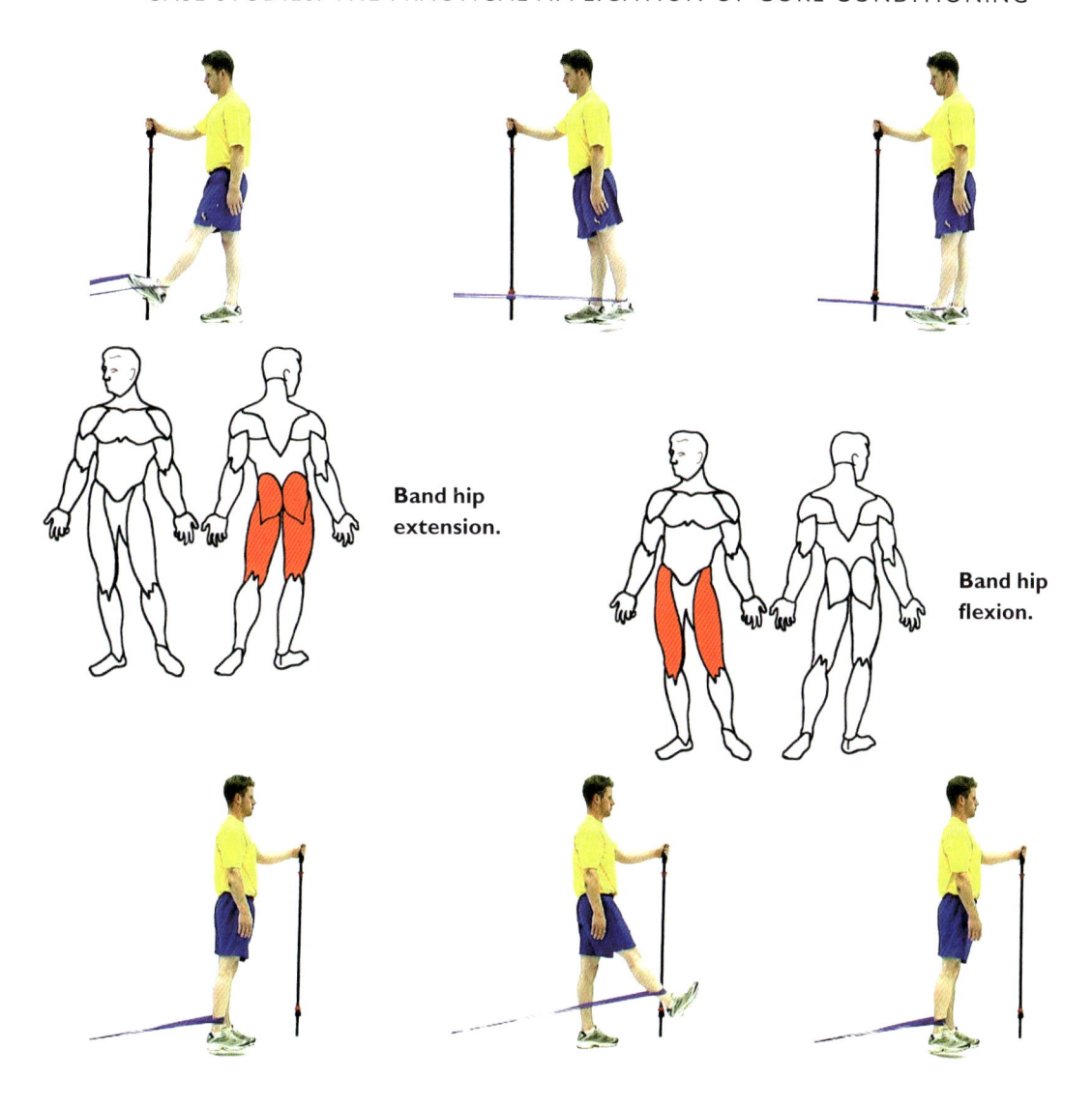

Band hip flexion.

- The amount of hip extension may be determined by the flexibility in the hip joint.

Caution: do not allow the lumbar spine to increase the neutral lordosis. Ensure that the band or tubing is securely attached.

HIP FLEXION CABLE ROTATION
Work at the same time as the extension/flexion exercise above.
3 x 12 L and R.

20 seconds rest in between each set.
When the quality goes, rest.

- Rotate the torso, pivot on the front foot and lift the knee in a running fashion.
- Dorsi flex the foot as the hip is flexed.
- The total range of movement may vary depending on flexibility of the hip.

Caution: ensure that the cable is securely attached to the lower leg. Do not round the shoulders or flex the spine during the exercise.

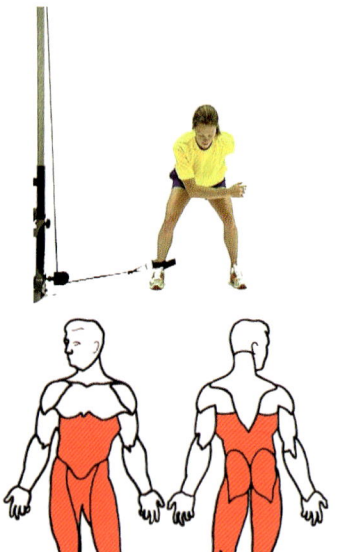

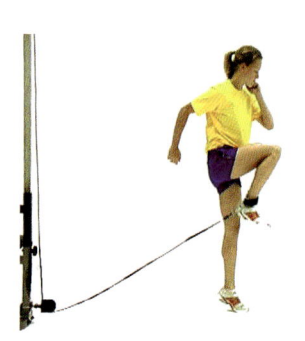

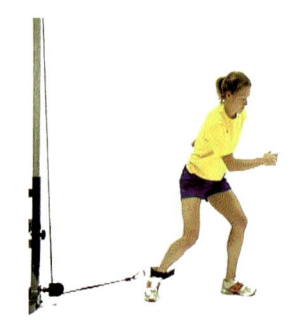

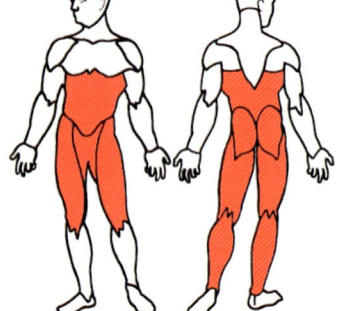

CASE STUDIES: THE PRACTICAL APPLICATION OF CORE CONDITIONING

Hip flexion cable rotation.

BOSU MEDICINE BALL ROTATION
(Sit on a cushion or balance cushion if no BOSU.) 30 second rotations x 4–5 repetitions. Feet off the floor.

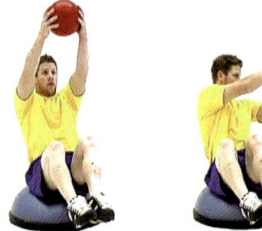

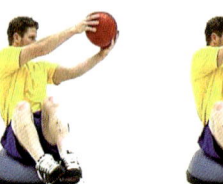

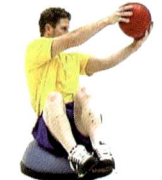

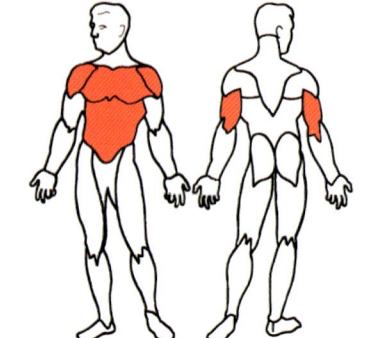

BOSU medicine ball rotation.

- Start with the feet off the ground and maintain tension in the torso throughout the exercise.
- Press the medicine ball to various positions with an emphasis on rotation.
- Keep the feet off the ground.
- 'Brace' your core throughout the movement.
- Dumbbells or a weights plate can be used as an alternative form of resistance.

Caution: take care not to fall backwards off the BOSU as the ball is pressed to various positions.

Additional/Supplementary Conditioning Exercises

Phase 1 = Weeks 1–8
Phase 2 = Weeks 9–16

Progressions

Exercises were progressed as follows:

- Increased load progression. Worked to body weight initially for confidence and progressed to add load in addition to increased repetitions where appropriate.
- Different planes of movement were progressed into the programme: the sports that the client wants to return to demand multi-directional capacity and reactive strength and also body contact.

CASE STUDIES: THE PRACTICAL APPLICATION OF CORE CONDITIONING

Exercise	Sets x reps and rest	Rationale	Comments
Phase 1 Supplementary Exercises: Weeks 1–8 Skipping (rope)	6 x 30 seconds 10 seconds rest in between each	Encourage dynamic control whilst extremities are moving: stretch-shortening/plyometric progression. As fatigue kicks in, maintain posture and control.	Double leg, single leg, LL, RR, etc., to add variation.
Lunge walk rotation	3 x 12 L and R side Strong rotation movement and good posture	Functional movement that demands good mobility and strength.	Progress from body weight to loaded with weight plate/medicine ball.
Stability ball single-leg squat	3 x 8 L and R Work alternate leg	Great for lower limb control: target = 90 degrees flexion. Stability in the pelvis, glutes, quads/hamstrings also good proprioceptive control.	Increased load well and good range of movement/depth achieved: quad parallel to the floor with limited accessory movement. Good control.
Multi-directional lunges (clock lunges) (4 points on the clock face)	3 x 4 rotations L and R x 3 sets (12 L and R per set) Work alternate leg 30 seconds rest between sets	Lower limb functional multi-directional movement. Good posture throughout the different lunge positions.	High volume. Minimal rest to improve endurance capacity and functional movement. Progress load.
Proprioception	4 x 20 seconds L and R leg Work alternate leg	Always an important addition to any rehab plan: encourage good posture, kicking ball, passing ball etc. during session.	Good adherence and improvement over time. Likes the involvement of a ball!
Phase 2 Supplementary Exercises: Weeks 9–16 Kettle bell swings	3 x 8 30 seconds rest in between sets	Encourage segmental control in a dynamic movement pattern. Triple flexion-triple extension movement pattern is highly functional and requires excellent core control.	Progressed range and load and explosiveness as confidence improved. Transfers into Gaelic football well.

- Decreased stability to increase the challenge: proprioception work was very important. Engaging the core and using tools, like a football, rugby ball, etc., to pass back, kick back and so on, were all encouraged and progressed. Dynamic proprioception was also introduced in the later stages, where hops from height, BOSU and mini trampoline hops and holds, different angles and so on, with control were introduced.

Exercise	Sets x reps and rest	Rationale	Comments
Dead lift	4 x 8 45 seconds rest in between	Good strength required in the upward and lowering phase through the lumbar spine. Important for strength and power progression and development. Triple flexion – triple extension.	The client enjoyed this as it provided a good 'feel' and sensation of loading. Progressed load well.
Double-leg bounding and diagonal bounding	3 x 8 jumps bounding. 3 x 8 jumps diagonal bounding. Walk back recovery on each.	Provide plyometric and stretch-shortening stimulus. Demand correct landing and take-off mechanics.	Able to progress from small bunny hops to larger, more demanding bounding/plyometric movement.
Proprioception: kept in the programme during Weeks 9–16.			

Progressions of exercise selection:

- Activities began in a controlled, isometric-based phase then progressed to more dynamic, concentric-eccentric work.
- Core work used cables and medicine balls to add complexity and challenge once the baseline control was established.
- The client was really enthused to add this challenge and felt that the demands placed upon him would allow him to become stronger and lead to a successful return to sport and full contact.

Outcome

- I saw the client on average once every week.
- It took a few weeks for the client to establish confidence as his pain reduced and function improved.
- Intensity RPE progressed from 4–5 (moderate to hard) to 7–8 (very hard–very, very hard) as confidence grew and strength improved. The client's capacity to work at a high intensity increased.
- Pain RPE was around 1–2 or zero over time.
- His adherence to the programme was very good, the client was determined to return to sport.
- He saw his physiotherapist in addition to seeing me, and we maintained good communication. Multi-disciplinary approach was good.
- His body awareness improved over the weeks.
- The whole level of function for this client improved: his low back pain reduced to zero and his level of resilience, strength and robustness was greatly improved as a result of the conditioning and rehabilitation programme. He returned to full-contact sport.

CASE STUDY 3

Assessment

Diagnosis: piriformis syndrome and associated muscle weakness. History of spinal fusion at L4-S1.

Definition:
The piriformis muscle is situated in the buttock near to the hip joint. Piriformis syndrome is a condition in which this muscle can develop spasm

CASE STUDIES: THE PRACTICAL APPLICATION OF CORE CONDITIONING

Needs Analysis

Client name	Client # 3
Occupation	Business Professional
DOB/age	42 years old
Sports/physical activities completed	Horse riding (4 x per week), cycle 8 miles to and from work (3 x per week), Pilates (1 x per week) Other training: CrossFit, running, triathlon, gym
Training history	Until recently was doing CrossFit but gradually ended up with very tight glutes/hamstrings/piriformis syndrome. Has since been seeing soft-tissue specialist and doing Pilates to strengthen core and learn to move correctly.
Injury history *Please include date of injury, surgical dates, investigations/scans, left/right side, etc. Please be as specific as possible.*	Assessment by sports medicine professional recommended strengthening posterior chain as glutes and hamstrings are especially weak. Had spinal fusion L4-S1 in 1996, which hasn't caused issues in itself, but over the years I have had to get my back functioning more normally as I had no rehab at the time. Recent MRI/x-ray showed no issues with discs/spine so can go ahead with training but adapted to avoid loading spine from above (barbell weighted squats etc.). Have had 3 occasions in recent years where think have strained SI joints leaving me unable to sit down on normal chairs for several weeks so have been trying to stretch hamstrings, glutes and mobilize back. Showing some progress. In summary I feel as if I over-use some muscles and under-use others and although I've focused on this in my training it hasn't really solved my issues. I need help to reduce pain and improve my strength!
Goals/training targets *e.g. stronger legs, leaner, general fitness improvement, upcoming events and dates*	Strengthen posterior chain and core. Gain freedom of movement through back and legs, reduce tightness and soreness, especially glutes/hamstrings.
Commitments *e.g. work, family, time constraints, etc.*	Work full time. Horse riding occupies a fair bit of spare time but have time for training.
Gym access and facilities	No gym membership at the moment. Have home-based equipment: Swiss ball, bands, rollers, basic weights at home and have reasonable awareness of training from using a personal trainer a few years ago.
Referring practitioner (if relevant)	Musculoskeletal Sports Physician
Any other relevant information	Driving and sitting on flights is quite an issue for me. I am hoping that getting stronger and more balanced in my movement will help with this.

or trigger points and cause pain in the buttock and referring down the back of the leg. Spasm in the piriformis muscle can also irritate the sciatic nerve, which lies close to it and even sometimes passes through the muscle. This can cause pain, numbness and tingling along the back of the leg and into the foot (http://www.gloshospitals.nhs.uk/en/Wards-and-Departments/Departments/Pain-Management/Different-Pains/Nerve-Pain/Types-of-Nerve-Pain/Nerve-Entrapment/Piriformis-Syndrome/).

Current presentation:
General day-to-day function is OK but client struggles with long duration of sitting and especially travel (flights and car journeys). Pain is experienced in glutes and sacroiliac joint, and hamstrings feel weak and tight. Client enjoys horse riding but seated position not very comfortable at present.

Exercise prescription:
Prescribed session to be completed 3 x each week.
Core strength work: 3–4 x each week.
Emphasis on quality of movement and attention to detail with prescribed movement patterns.

Other things to consider:
Targets:

- Improve mobility: thoracic spine and lumbar spine.
- Posterior chain strength improvement.
- Introduce regular myofascial release work, specifically ITB, glutes, lumbar spine.

Challenges/concerns:
Client aware of axial loading due to history of spinal fusion at L4-S1 in 1996. Recent MRI indicates that there is a stable Grade I spondylolisthesis of L5 on S1 to be aware of with loading plan.
  Needs to get stronger.

Strength and Conditioning Plan

Checklist:

- Ensure excellent understanding of exercises and positions and build confidence for loading patterns.
- Body awareness and positioning when completing exercise needs to be excellent.
- Attention to detail: breathing, bracing when moving, increasing load, regular myofascial release and mobility work.

Frequency:

- Core strength programme to be completed 3–4 x each week.
- Supplementary exercises to be completed 3 x each week.
- Mobility and myofascial release: daily.

Session duration:
Core strength and posterior chain = 40 minutes
Supplementary exercises = 20 minutes

Intensity:
Borg Rating of Perceived Exertion (RPE) = 4–5 (moderate–hard)
Target pain scale: <2–3 (easy–moderate) (Borg RPE used for pain scale)

Note to client:

- All exercises should be completed with absolute attention to detail and with excellent technique.
- 'Brace' position through your core, position of strength and belly breath to activate your muscles.
- If the quality of movement is compromised or things become sloppy because of fatigue, rest and then go again.
- Work on your body awareness and know where you should feel the muscles work.

CASE STUDIES: THE PRACTICAL APPLICATION OF CORE CONDITIONING

Core and Posterior Chain Strengthening Plan

- Complete the exercises 3–4 times each week, in addition to the prescribed additional reconditioning programme.
- Before every session, spinal mobility work (see table) to be part of the daily routine.

Spinal Mobility

Exercise	Sets	Reps
Lumbar rolls	2	x 10 L and R
Lumbar rotations	2	x 10 L and R
Cat stretch and downward dog	2	3 blocks of 3 movement cycles = 1 set
Back extension	2	x 10
Seated slumps	3	x 8 L and R

Myofascial release:
Glutes, ITB, lumbar region (muscular area), 2 x 45 seconds on each area as follows:

Glute Self-Massage

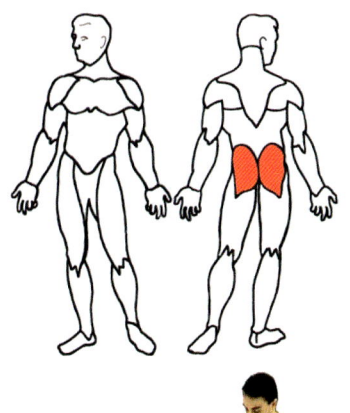

Glute self-massage.

- Place the foot on opposite knee and roll the buttock back and forth on the ball.
- Rotate the hips to massage all aspects of the buttocks.
- If a tight area is identified, pause and maintain pressure for a short period of time.

ITB SELF-MASSAGE
- Position the outside of the thigh on the ball with the leg straight.
- Roll forward and back over the ball, flexing the knee to increase the stretch.
- Roll from the hip all the way down the length of the thigh and rotate the leg to vary the location of the massage.
- If a tight area is identified, pause and maintain pressure for a short period of time.

STANDING SPINAL SELF-MASSAGE
- Place a ball against the wall and against the paraspinal muscles.
- Squat up and down continuously to roll the back muscles against the ball. Vary the position of the ball to change the emphasis on the muscles being massaged.
- You may need to reposition the ball if it moves out of position. If a tight area is identified, pause and maintain pressure for a short period of time.

Different balls and other implements can be used to perform the self-massage.

Caution: take care rolling the ball around bony structures, particularly around the spine. A slight discomfort may be experienced but do not apply pressure to the point of pain.

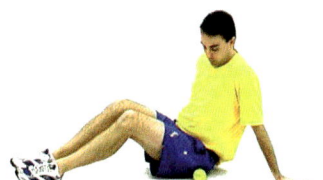

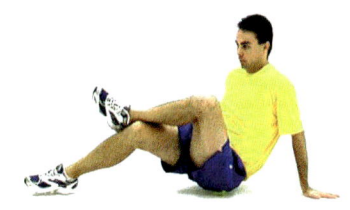

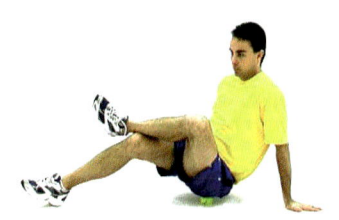

CASE STUDIES: THE PRACTICAL APPLICATION OF CORE CONDITIONING

ITB self-massage.

- Increase the length of the steps or decrease the contact time with the ground to modify the exercise.
- Vary the angles and movement patterns to activate the glutes.

Caution: ensure the band is secure and strong enough to withstand the tension developed during this exercise.

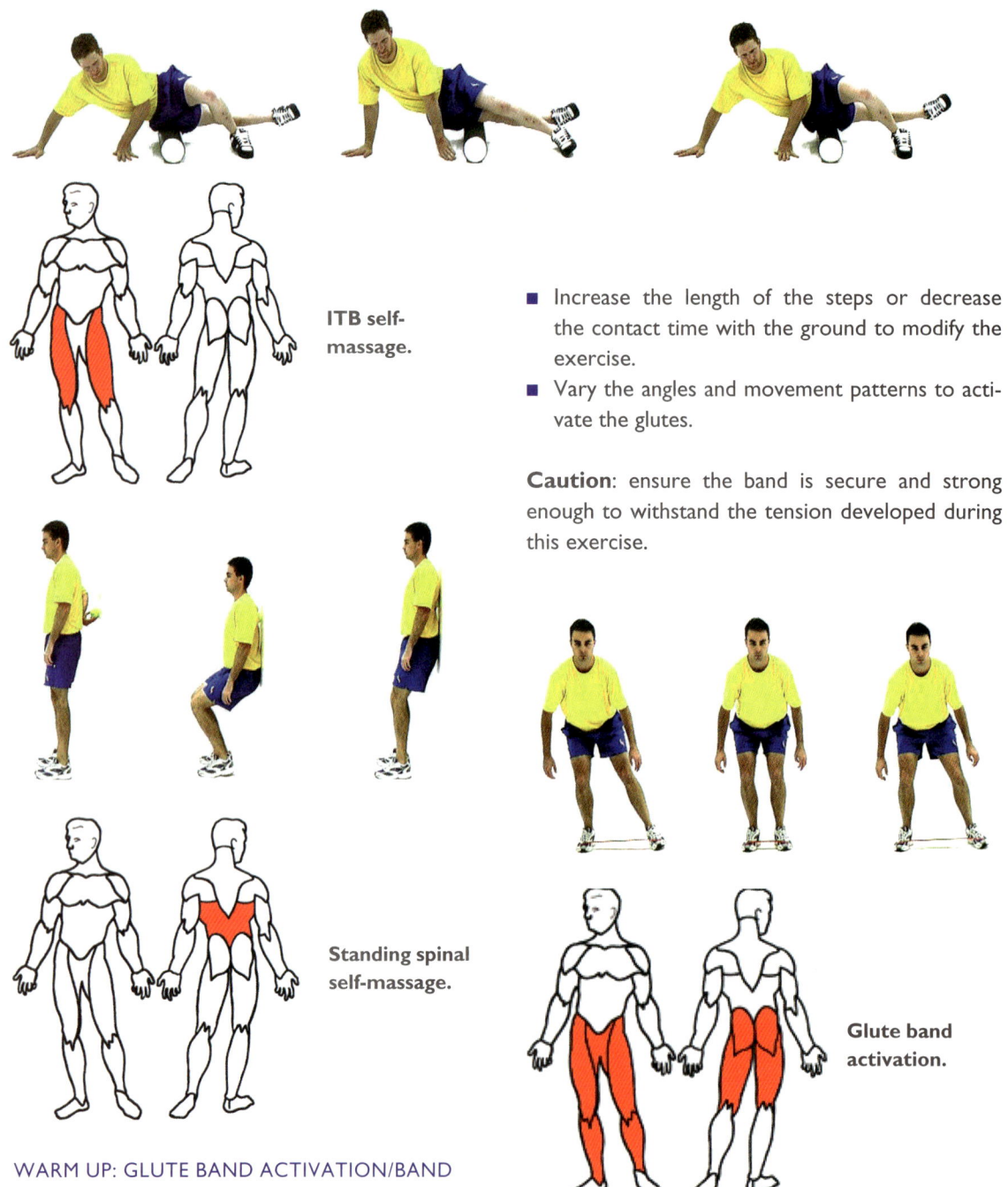

Standing spinal self-massage.

Glute band activation.

WARM UP: GLUTE BAND ACTIVATION/BAND WALKS

Complete 3 sets left and right to fatigue.

- Secure the band around the feet and walk sideways and diagonally whilst maintaining the tension of the band.

SINGLE-LEG BRIDGING

3 x 8 left and right side.
Work alternate leg.

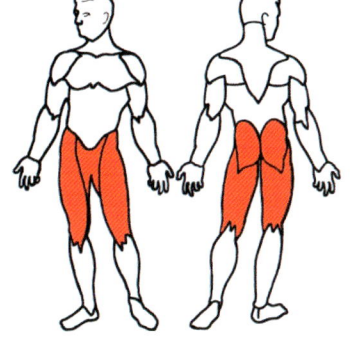

CASE STUDIES: THE PRACTICAL APPLICATION OF CORE CONDITIONING

- Hold for 2–3 seconds, and then control the movements back to the start position.

STRAIGHT LEG/ROMANIAN DEAD LIFT

4 × 8 repetitions.
30 seconds rest in between.

- Assume a parallel stance with the hands wide on the barbell.
- Begin with the bar close to the shins with the arms straight and the shoulders over the bar.
- Keep the chest up and look forward or slightly up, with neutral curves in the spine.
- Flex at the hips until the bar travels below the knees then extend the hips to reverse the movement back to the start position.
- Complete the prescribed number of sets and repetitions

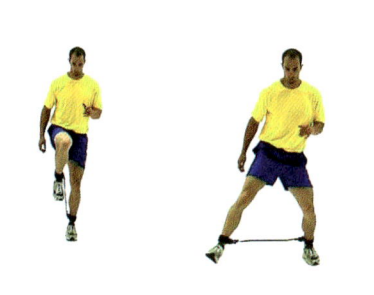

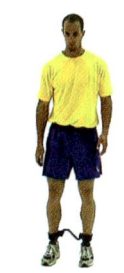

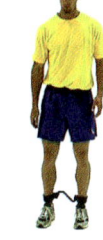

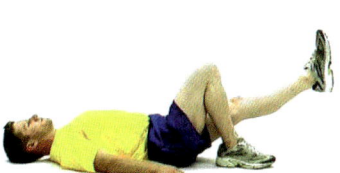

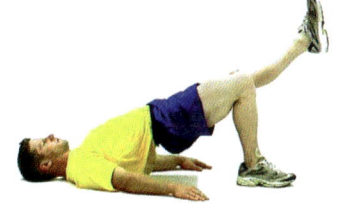

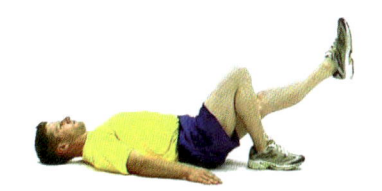

Band walks.

Caution: do not flex the spine or allow the shoulders to round. Do not allow the hips to rise before the shoulders.

SWISS BALL CURLS

3 sets of 6–8 repetitions.
Work alternate leg. Rest if the quality is compromised.

- Position the feet securely on the stability ball with the hands on the floor.
- Lift the hips off the floor until the legs are in line with the torso then flex the legs to bring the ball towards the hips.
- Return back to the start position with both legs.
- Vary the position of the hands on the floor to assist with balance and place the hands across the chest to progress the difficulty of the exercise.

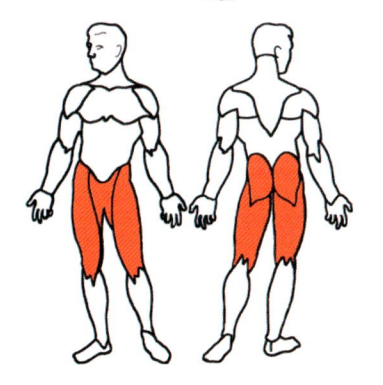

Single-leg bridging.

- Start with the feet approximately shoulder width apart with the head and shoulders in contact with the ground.
- Lift the hips off the ground until the thighs are in line with the torso.
- Then lift one leg up and straight out, in line with your body.

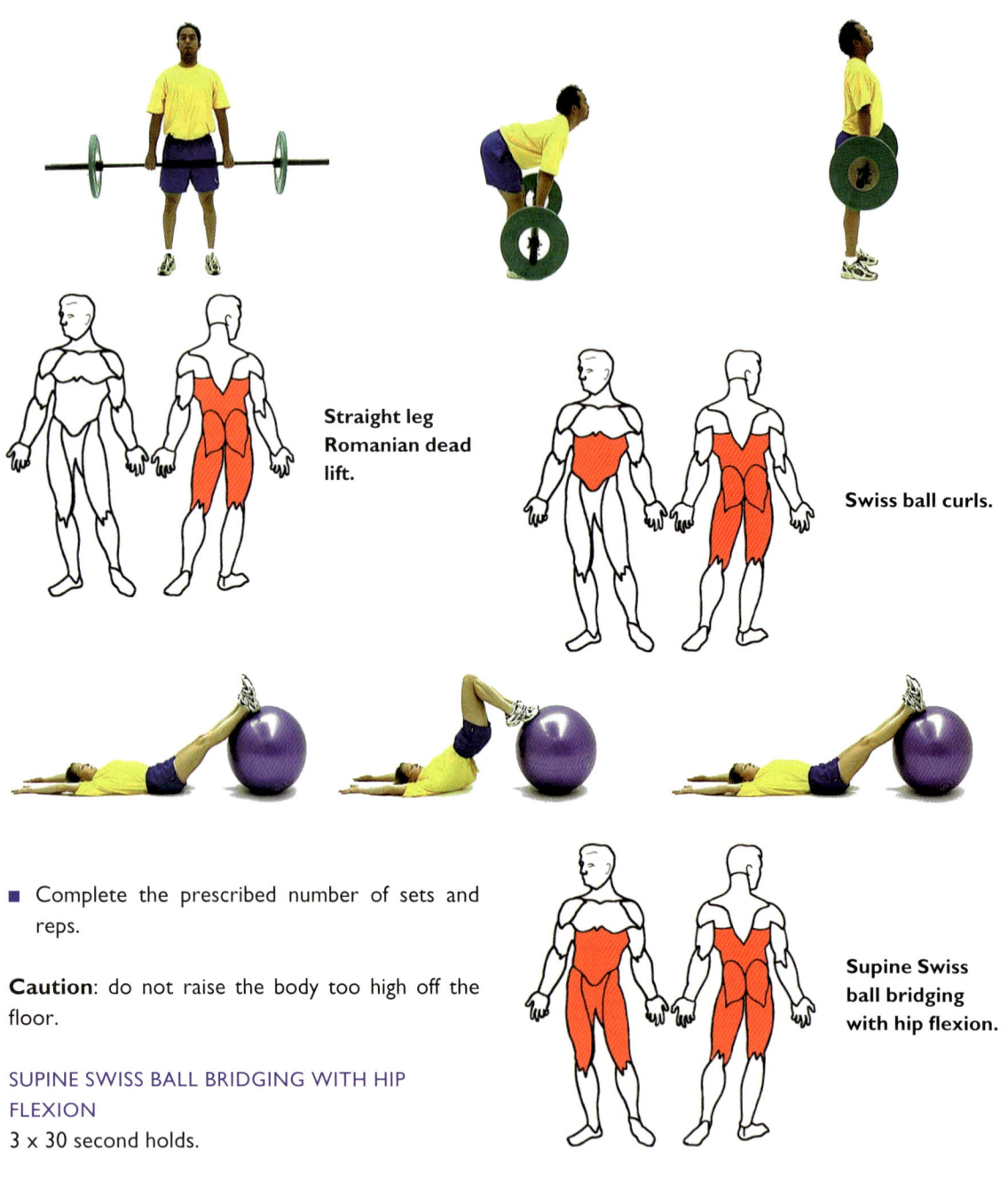

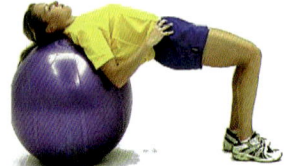

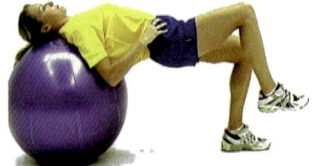

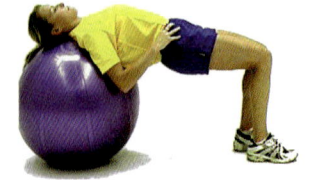

CASE STUDIES: THE PRACTICAL APPLICATION OF CORE CONDITIONING

Straight leg Romanian dead lift.

Swiss ball curls.

- Complete the prescribed number of sets and reps.

Caution: do not raise the body too high off the floor.

Supine Swiss ball bridging with hip flexion.

SUPINE SWISS BALL BRIDGING WITH HIP FLEXION
3 x 30 second holds.

CASE STUDIES: THE PRACTICAL APPLICATION OF CORE CONDITIONING

Progressing to 3 x 10 repetitions left and right, hold each raise/rep for 3–4 seconds. Belly breathe and brace as you lift.

- Start with the head and shoulders on the stability ball with the knees in line with the hips and the feet under the knees.
- Maintain the bridging position for the prescribed duration.
- Progression: lift one foot off the ground then place it back on to the ground. Hold for 2–3 seconds.
- Repeat the movements with alternate legs continuously with excellent control.
- Place the hands across the chest, out wide or above the head while maintaining the same body position to vary and progress the exercise.

Caution: maintain a neutral spine and level pelvic position and do not allow the lower back to excessively extend.

SINGLE-LEG SPLIT GOOD MORNING EXERCISE
(*Unlike the image, place the load in front as in the Romanian dead lift. Use a weight plate across the chest, for example.*)
3 x 8 left and right leg.
Work alternate leg.

- Start with one leg straight and the other leg slightly flexed in a split position (slightly longer than the image).
- You can also raise the front leg on a bench/step to increase the sensation.
- Hold the load in front of you whilst maintaining a straight/flat back with neutral spine.
- Lean forward, tilting at the hips while maintaining neutral spinal curves.
- Keep the chest up and continue to look forward or slightly up.
- The load should stay in line with your body: do not move away as this will put additional pressure on the spine.

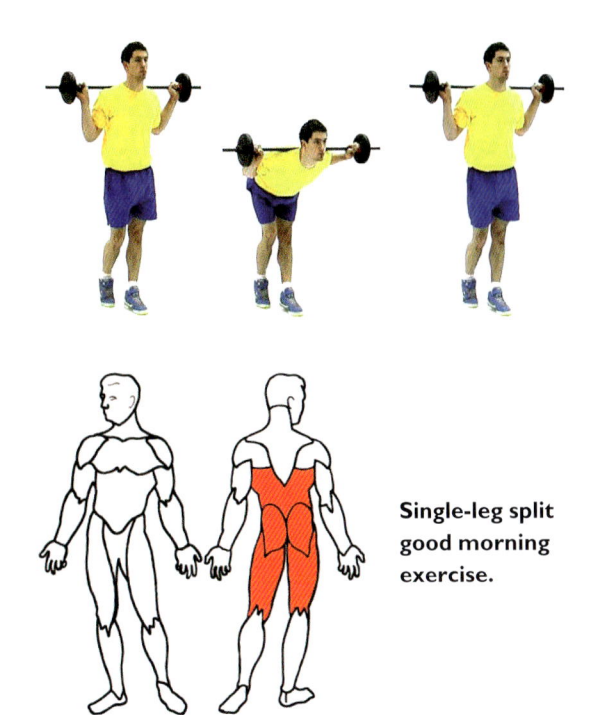

Single-leg split good morning exercise.

- Slowly lower, tilting forwards until you feel your hamstrings on the straight (forward) leg and then slowly return to the starting position.
- Speed of movement: count of 4 down, 1 transition and 2 back.

Caution: do not round the spine.

BOSU SUPINE ISOMETRIC STABILIZATION
4 x 15–20 second isometric holds.
Progress duration as strength improves.
5–10 seconds rest in between each set.

- Start with the low back supported on the BOSU and the shoulders and head unsupported.
- The torso should be either straight or slightly flexed.
- Take both feet off the ground and hold the position for the prescribed time.
- Activate your pelvic floor muscle as you hold, breathe and brace in the isometric hold position.

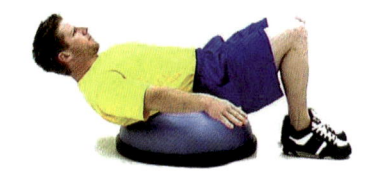

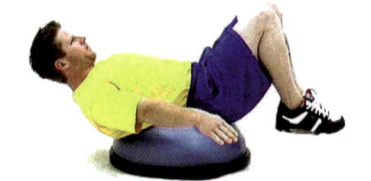

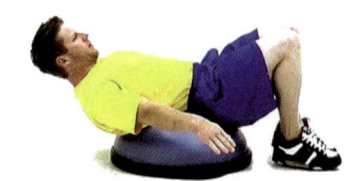

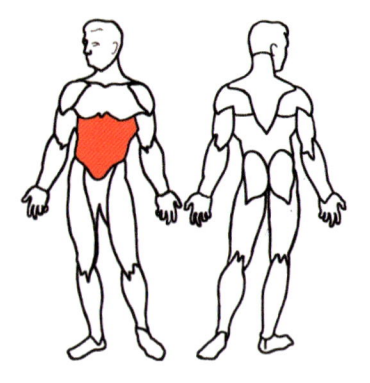

CASE STUDIES: THE PRACTICAL APPLICATION OF CORE CONDITIONING

BOSU supine isometric stabilization.

Caution: keep the neck in line with the spine and the hands wide for balance.

PRONE HIP EXTENSION

3 x 8 repetitions.
30 seconds rest in between each set.

- Start with the hips over the pad and keep the upper body stationary.
- Extend the hips upwards then slowly return the legs to the start position.
- Complete the prescribed number of sets and reps with excellent technique and control.

Caution: keep the neck in line with the spine. Do not extend the legs past the level of the body.

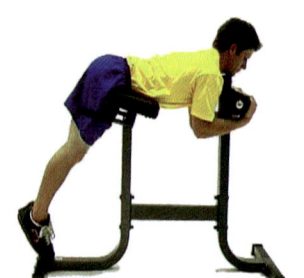

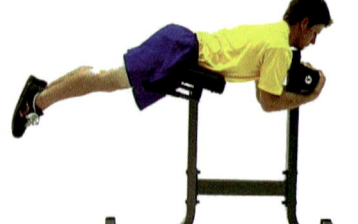

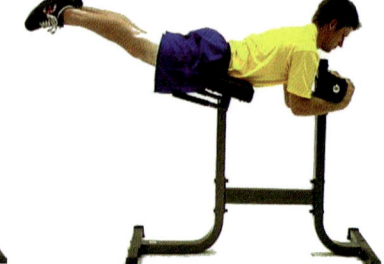

HIP ROTATION: INTERNAL AND EXTERNAL ROTATION

Complete 3 sets of 8–10 internal/external rotations. Work alternate leg.

- Start with the hip flexed to approximately 90 degrees.
- Maintaining the same horizontal position of the thigh, internally and externally rotate the hip.
- Gradually increase the range as the mobility of the hip improves.

Caution: the movements should be at the hips and not the spine. Discontinue the stretch if pain or discomfort is experienced in the hip joint.

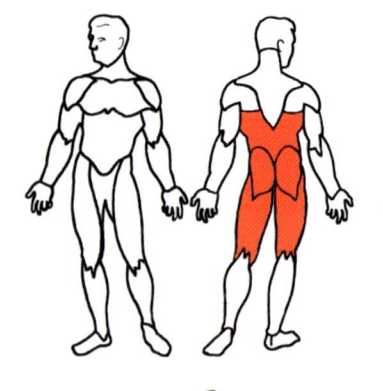

Prone hip extension.

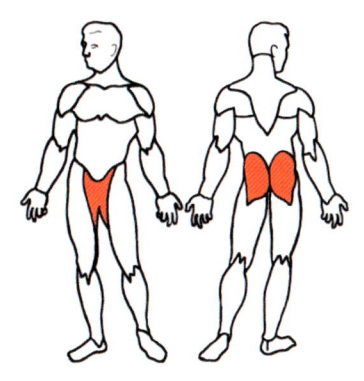

CASE STUDIES: THE PRACTICAL APPLICATION OF CORE CONDITIONING

- The duration of the stretch should be short; repeat the process.

Caution: keep the head and shoulders relaxed and in contact with the ground.

HIP INTERNAL ROTATION STRETCH

2 x 6–8 L and R side.
Use a band or hands to assist.

- Keep the thigh perpendicular to the ground and place the other hand on the knee to stabilize the leg.
- Internally rotate the hip and pull further to increase the stretch as the internal rotator muscles continue to contract.
- The duration of the stretch should be short; repeat the process.

Caution: keep the head and shoulders relaxed and in contact with the ground.

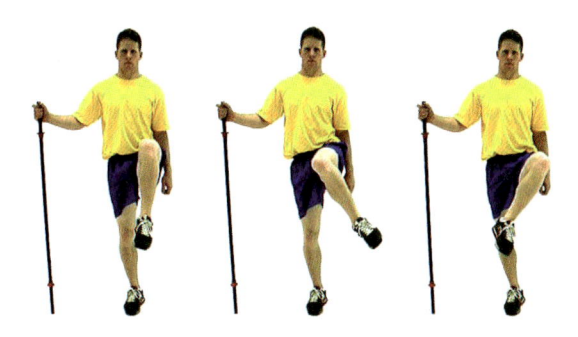

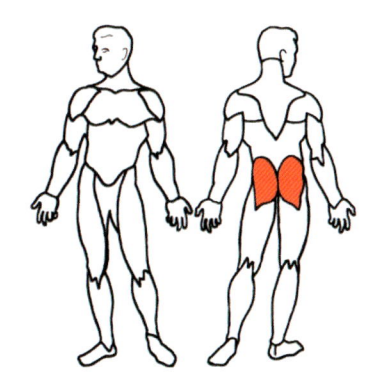

Hip rotation: internal and external rotation.

HIP EXTERNAL ROTATION STRETCH

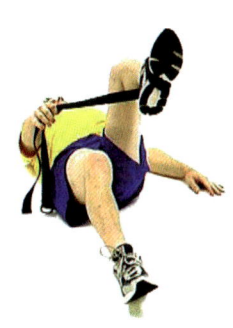

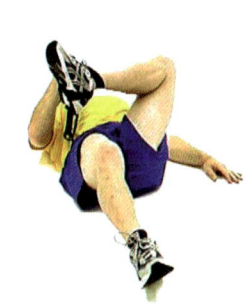

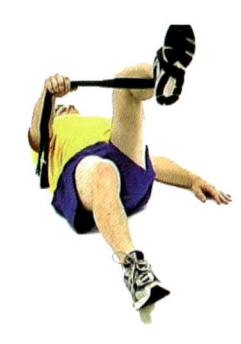

2 x 6–8 L and R side.
Use a band or hands to assist.

- Keep the thigh perpendicular to the ground and place the other hand on the knee to stabilize the leg if need be.
- Externally rotate the hip and pull further to increase the stretch as the external rotator muscles continue.

Hip external rotation stretch.

73

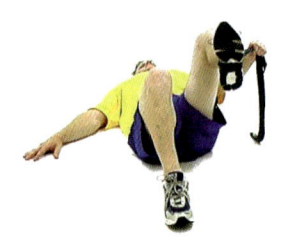

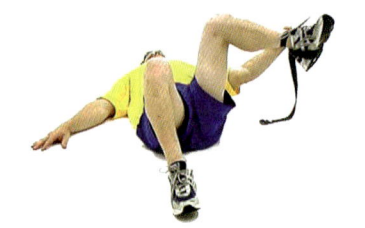

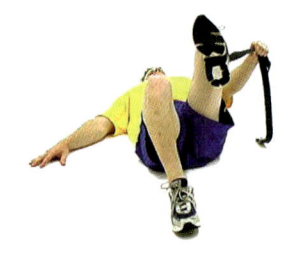

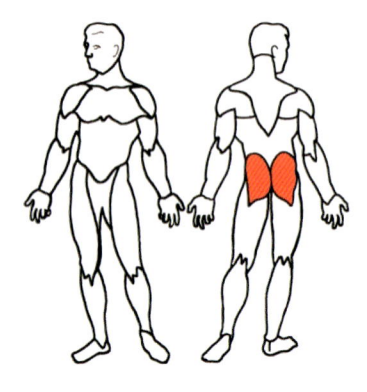

CASE STUDIES: THE PRACTICAL APPLICATION OF CORE CONDITIONING

Hip internal rotation stretch.

Additional/Supplementary Conditioning Exercises

Progressions

Exercises were progressed as follows:

- Increased load progression: worked to body weight initially for confidence and progressed to add load in addition to increased repetitions

Exercise	Sets x reps and rest	Rationale	Comments
Split squat	3 x 12 L and R Work alternate leg (no rest)	Good lower limb strengthening.	Found hard initially but progressed to load by week 2.
Bent-over row	4 x 8 reps 30 seconds rest in between	Good low back strengthening exercise. Bent knee position and strong back provide a good point of stability and trunk strength.	Loaded with dumbbells initially. Progress to barbell. Excellent movement pattern and strength/position. Likes the feel of the load.
Stability ball single-leg squat	3 x 8 L and R Work alternate leg	Great for lower limb control: target = 90 degrees flexion. Stability in the pelvis, glutes, quads/hamstrings also good proprioceptive control. Will hopefully transfer into strength benefit when riding.	Good range of movement/depth achieved: quad parallel to the floor with limited accessory movement. Good control. Progressed to load by week 3.
Proprioception	4 x 20 seconds L and R leg Work alternate leg	Always an important addition to any rehab plan: encourage good posture, kicking ball, passing ball, etc., during session.	Good adherence and improvement over time.
Dead lift	4 x 8 45 seconds rest in between	Good strength required in the upward and lowering phase through the lumbar spine. Important for strength and power progression and development.	The client was nervous to begin with, but increased confidence and felt good with loading as provided a good 'feel' of strength.

where appropriate. Double-leg Swiss ball curls progressed to single-leg over time, BOSU supine isometric stabilization progressed to more dynamic movements, moving the legs as the client became stronger. Dead lift, Romanian dead lift and single-leg good morning with front load all increased load progression.

Progressions of exercise selection:

- Activities began in a controlled, isometric-based phase or slow and controlled eccentric work and then progressed over time to more dynamic movements.
- Hip mobility was important to help release the piriformis and improve hip and lumbar spine mobility, which helped to off-load the demand placed on the hamstrings. This had a very positive effect on the client's pain whilst seated: a big improvement reducing pain to zero after 4 weeks.
- The spinal mobility, slumps and myofascial release were completed in general 5 x each week and really helped.

Outcome

- I saw the client on average once every 3 weeks.
- The client's body awareness was very good as she had a good training history.
- The client was able to increase the session intensity RPE quite quickly, progressing from an initial prescription of 4–5 (moderate to hard) to 7–8 (very hard to very, very hard) as her strength improved and pain reduced: the client's capacity to work at a high intensity increased.
- Pain RPE was around 1 or zero over time and improved significantly with long journeys and horse riding.
- Pelvic control was much better and horse riding was now pain-free. The client felt strong.
- Postural control was improved as well as general strength.

- The combination of increased strength and improved mobility and muscle release worked together, resulting in a very positive outcome.

CASE STUDY 4

Assessment

Diagnosis: bilateral hamstring tendinopathy with some para-tendinitis. History of low back pain and pelvic floor problems post-partum.

Definition:
Hamstring tendonitis is inflammation of the hamstring tendon as it attaches to the ischial tuberosity at the top of the back of the thigh. It can follow a tear of the hamstring tendon that is poorly treated or more often is an over-use injury (http://www.sportsinjuryclinic.net/sport-injuries/thigh-pain/back-thigh/hamstring-origin-tendonitis).

Paratenonitis (inflammation of the paratenon) occurs when a tendon rubs excessively over a bony protuberance. The increased friction results in inflammation (Khan *et al.*, 1999).

Pelvic floor dysfunction: the pelvic floor is a sheet of muscle through which the rectum passes and becomes the anal canal. The anal canal is surrounded by the anal sphincter complex, which is comprised of both an internal and external component. In addition to the rectum, the urethra, which carries urine from the bladder to the outside of the body, also passes through the front portion of the pelvic floor, as does the vagina in females. Improper functioning of the pelvic floor muscles can cause a number of specific conditions and disorders (American Society of Colon and Rectal Surgeons, https://www.fascrs.org/patients/disease-condition/pelvic-floor-dysfunction-expanded-version).

Current presentation:
Onset of pain when jogging/running. No other daily pain.

CASE STUDIES: THE PRACTICAL APPLICATION OF CORE CONDITIONING

Needs Analysis

Client name	Client # 4
Occupation	Housewife
DOB/age	42 years old
Sports/physical activities completed	Running, gym work, weekly Pilates class
Training history	I ran a marathon in 2005 and have done some 10k runs since. I had my first child in 2006 and my second (by Caesarean) in 2008 and have continued to exercise regularly but at a reduced level.
Injury history *Please include date of injury, surgical dates, investigations/ scans, left/right side, etc. Please be as specific as possible.*	In the last two years I have been seeing a physio for back pain (and pelvic floor problems) but this has largely subsided. However, in about April of this year I developed pain in my hamstrings when I ran, which was initially treated as hamstring strain by my physio. On the recommendation of my physio I recently saw a sports medicine physician and he requested an MRI, which confirmed that I have bilateral hamstring tendinopathy with some paratenonitis. He has recommended that I stop running and work on strengthening my legs. I don't feel much discomfort/pain unless I jog or run.
Goals/training targets *e.g. stronger legs, leaner, general fitness improvement, upcoming events and dates*	I would like to be able to run without discomfort for at least 30 minutes, ideally I would like to run for up to an hour.
Commitments *e.g. work, family, time constraints, etc.*	I have two young children (4 and 6 years) who are at school between 8.50am and 3.20pm – I prefer to exercise whilst they are at school.
Gym access and facilities	I am a member of a gym.
Referring practitioner (if relevant)	Musculoskeletal Sports Physician
Any other relevant information	Nil

Exercise prescription:

- Prescribed session to be completed 3 x each week. This includes core, glute pelvic work in addition to specific hamstring/posterior chain and lower body loading.
- Emphasis on quality of movement and attention to detail with prescribed movement patterns.

Other things to consider:
Targets:

- Posterior chain strength improvement.
- Introduce regular myofascial release work specifically ITB, glutes and hamstrings.

CASE STUDIES: THE PRACTICAL APPLICATION OF CORE CONDITIONING

Challenges/concerns:

- History of low back pain and pelvic pain in addition to running history and hamstring tendinopathy may all be linked.

Strength and Conditioning Plan

Checklist:

- Prescribe a global plan: address hamstring tendinopathy within loading plan.
- Address glute and pelvic activation within programme.
- Strengthen core and functional movement specifically for running.

Frequency:

- Strength and conditioning programme to be completed 3 x each week.
- Mobility and myofascial release: 5 x each week.

Session duration:
Strength programme including core and posterior chain = 45–60 minutes

Intensity:
Borg Rating of Perceived Exertion (RPE) = 4–5 (moderate–hard).
Target pain scale: <2–3 (easy–moderate) (Borg RPE used for pain scale). Pain expected on eccentric loading, just not any higher than 3.

Note to client:

- All exercises should be completed with absolute attention to detail and with excellent technique.
- Pain on and also after eccentric work (DOMS) is to be anticipated as the client's tendinopathy is very acute. It is important that the client is aware of this and knows that they need to get through this to turn a corner in their rehabilitation, ensure that they achieve some tissue adaptation and progress.
- Reassure client that loading and pain is therefore acceptable.
- Activate pelvic floor muscles as you complete the exercises.
- Work on your body awareness and know where you should feel the muscles work.

Core and Posterior Chain Strengthening Plan

- Complete the exercises below 3 times each week.
- Before every session and 5 x each week, do spinal mobility work (see table).

Spinal Mobility

Exercise	Sets	Reps
Lumbar rolls	2	x 10 L and R
Lumbar rotations	2	x 10 L and R
Cat stretch and downward dog	2	3 blocks of 3 = 1 set
Back extension	2	x 10
Seated slumps	3	x 8 L and R

Myofascial release for glutes, ITB, hamstrings, quadriceps, calves:
Move the foam roller or tennis ball around the particular body part until you feel some discomfort. This is the trigger point! Hold the foam roller or tennis ball there until the muscle relaxes. This may take up to 30–45 seconds or until the muscle has relaxed and the pain has gone. Resume rolling until you find another trigger point. Stop and hold again until the pain goes. A treatment can take as long as you want; usually between 5 and 10 minutes is sufficient. Pre-session can be quicker but please make time to conduct longer sessions through the week.

CASE STUDIES: THE PRACTICAL APPLICATION OF CORE CONDITIONING

Work on each muscle group for 45 seconds up and down the muscle x 2 on each limb (L and R).

HAMSTRING SELF-MASSAGE
- Place one leg over the other and roll the posterior thigh back and forth on the foam roller or tennis ball, keeping the leg straight.
- Turn the thigh in and out to massage all aspects of the hamstrings.
- If a tight area is identified, pause and maintain pressure for a short period of time.

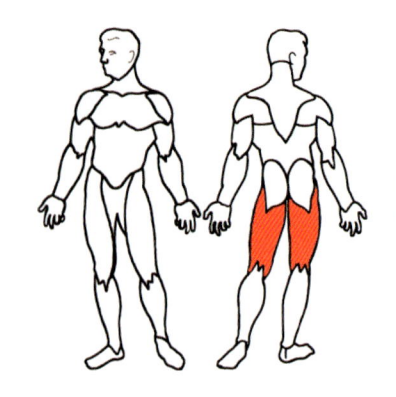

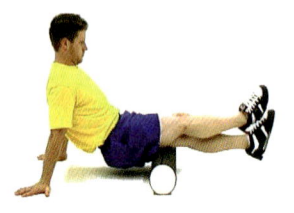

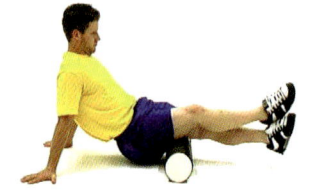

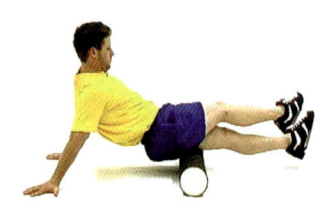

Hamstring self-massage.

QUAD SELF-MASSAGE
- Keep the forearms flat on the ground with the spine straight.
- Press the body forward and back against the ground to roll the front of the thighs over the roller.
- If a tight area is identified, pause and maintain pressure for a short period of time.

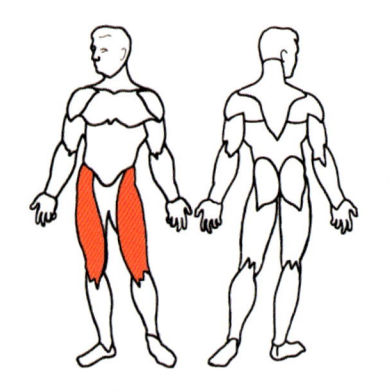

Quad self-massage.

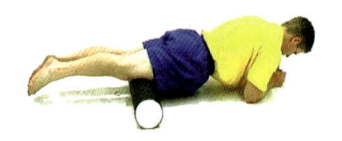

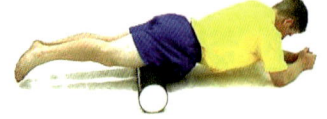

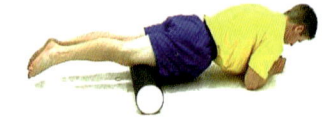

GLUTE SELF-MASSAGE
- Place the foot on the opposite knee and roll the buttock back and forth on the ball.
- Rotate the hips to massage all aspects of the buttocks.
- If a tight area is identified, pause and maintain pressure for a short period of time.

CALF SELF-MASSAGE
- Place one leg over the other and roll the calf muscle back and forth on the foam roller or tennis ball, keeping the leg straight.
- Turn the thigh in and out to massage all aspects of the calf.
- If a tight area is identified, pause and maintain pressure for a short period of time.

CASE STUDIES: THE PRACTICAL APPLICATION OF CORE CONDITIONING

Glute self-massage.

Calf self-massage.

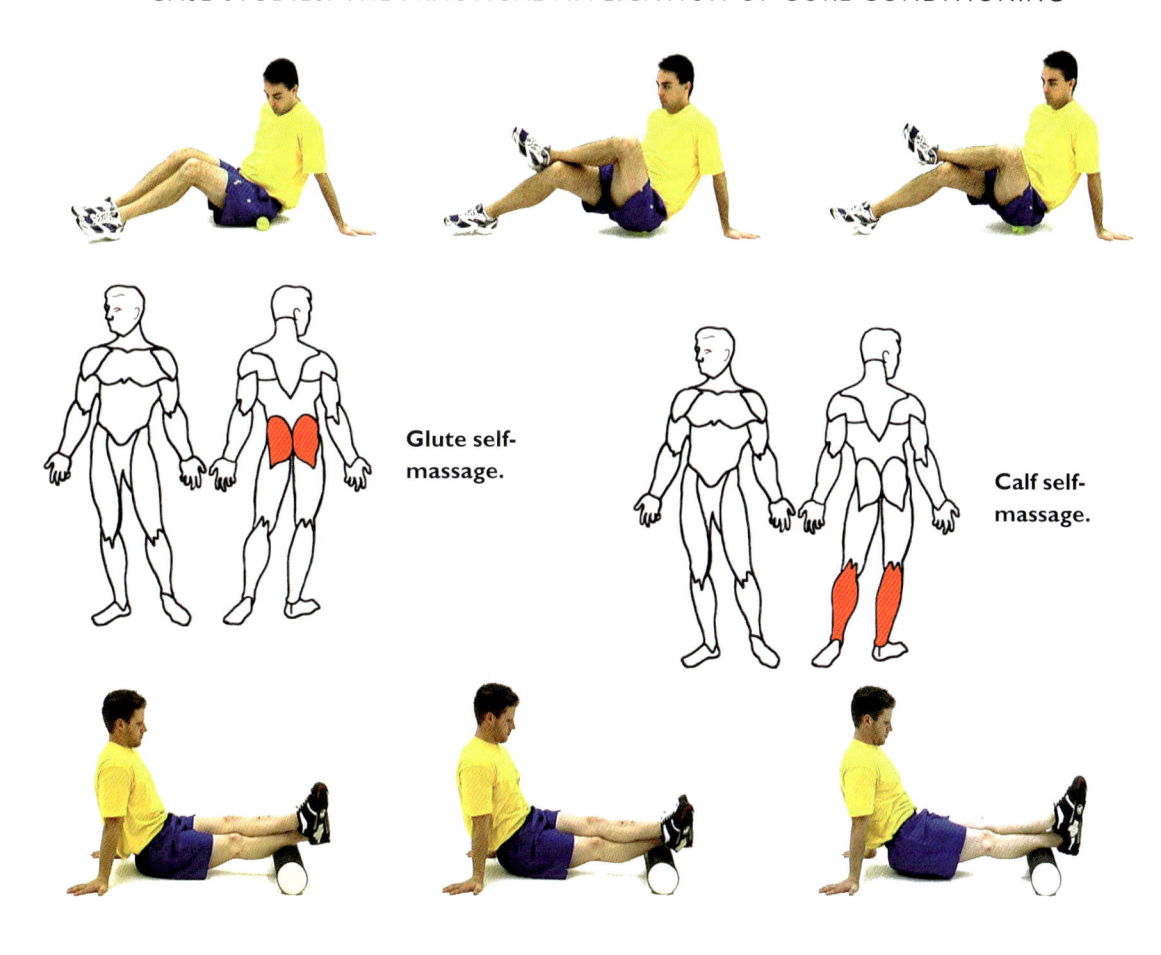

ITB SELF-MASSAGE
- Position the outside of the thigh on the ball with the leg straight.
- Roll forward and back over the ball, flexing the knee to increase the stretch.
- Roll from the hip all the way down the length of the thigh and rotate the leg to vary the location of the massage.
- If a tight area is identified, pause and maintain pressure for a short period of time.

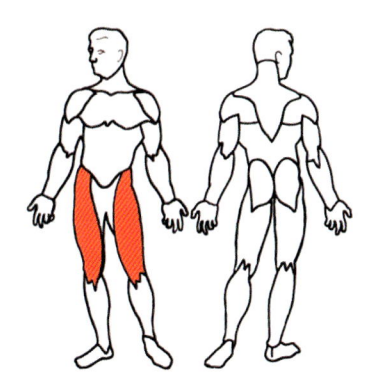

ITB self-massage.

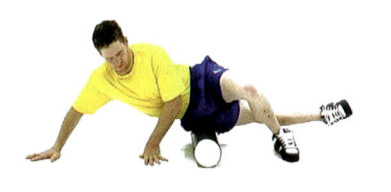

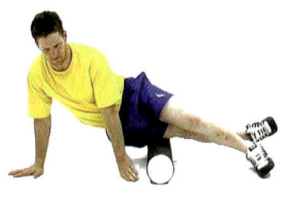

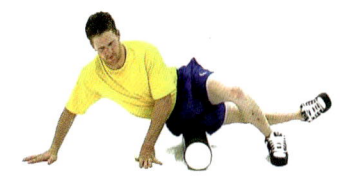

CASE STUDIES: THE PRACTICAL APPLICATION OF CORE CONDITIONING

Strength and Conditioning Programme

Complete 3 x each week.

GLUTE BAND ACTIVATION: BACKWARD WALKING

- 3 x left and right to fatigue.
- 5 seconds rest in between each set.

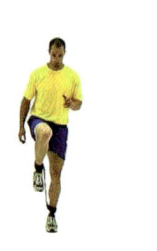

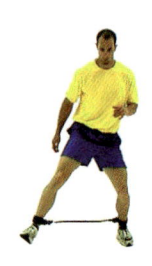

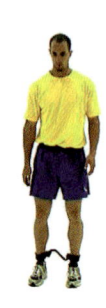

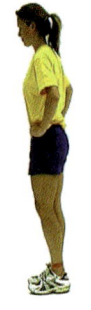

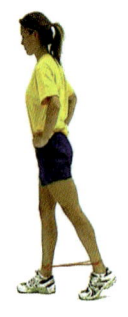

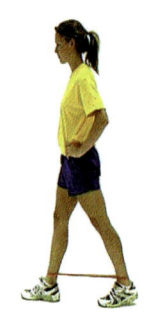

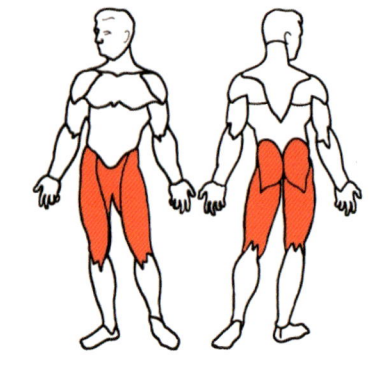

Band diagonal lunge walk.

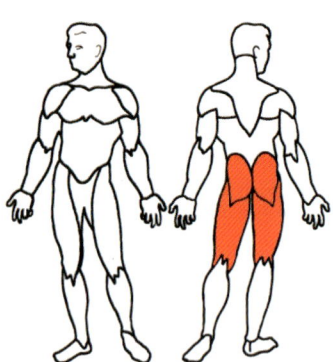

Glute band activation: backward walking.

BAND HIP ABDUCTION

- 3 x left and right to fatigue (stay on same side for fatigue/overload) then swap over.
- 5 seconds rest in between each set.

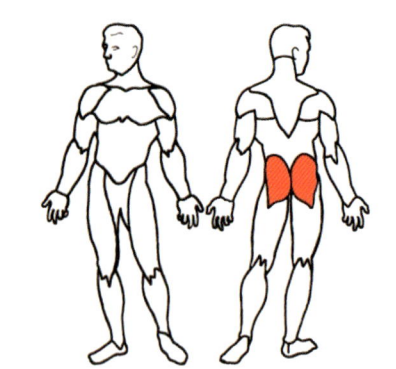

Band hip abduction.

BAND DIAGONAL LUNGE WALK

- Excellent technique.
- Band as load/resistance.
- Complete 3 x 8 left and right side.
- 5 seconds rest in between sets.

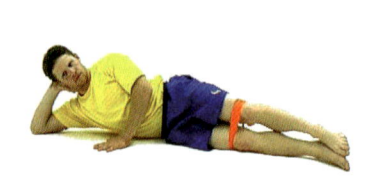

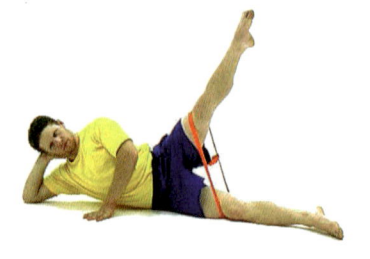

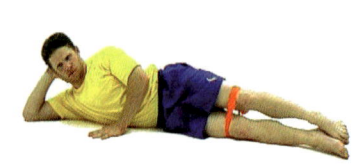

CASE STUDIES: THE PRACTICAL APPLICATION OF CORE CONDITIONING

SINGLE-LEG BRIDGING ON BENCH OR SWISS BALL

3 x 8 repetitions left and right, hold each raise/rep for 3 seconds.
Work alternate leg.

- Start with the feet approximately shoulder width apart with the head and shoulders in contact with the ground.
- Place your feet on the bench or Swiss ball.
- Lift the hips off the ground until the thighs are in line with the torso.

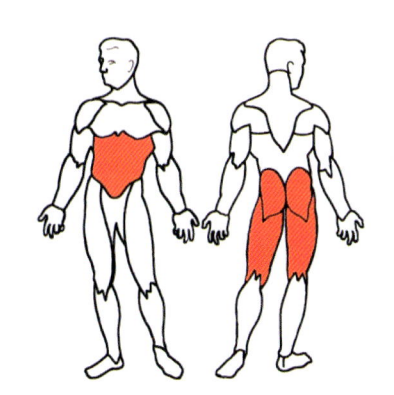

Single-leg bridging on bench or Swiss ball.

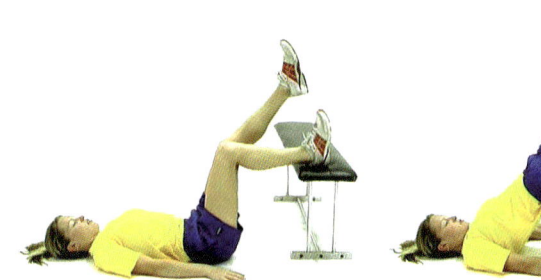

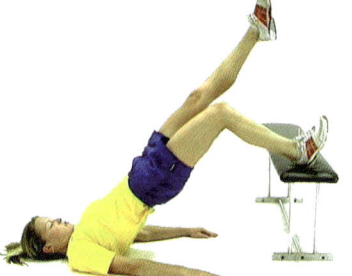

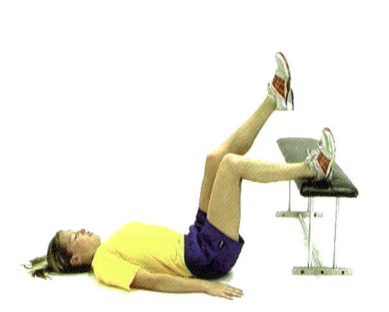

- Lift one leg up and straight out, in line with your body.
- Hold for 3 seconds, contract your pelvic floor and complete a belly breath and brace.
- Control the movement back to the start position.
- Complete the prescribed number of repetitions then swap legs.
- Breathe throughout the exercise especially as you raise your torso.
- Activate your pelvic floor as you lift and hold.

SINGLE-LEG STEP-UP: FRONT AND LATERAL

3 x 12 left and right-side front.
3 x 12 left and right-side lateral.
Work alternate leg: no rest.
Maintain quality of movement.
Activate pelvic floor during the exercise.

- Complete with body weight to start with.
- Face the box for front step-ups and start side-on for lateral step-ups (see image).

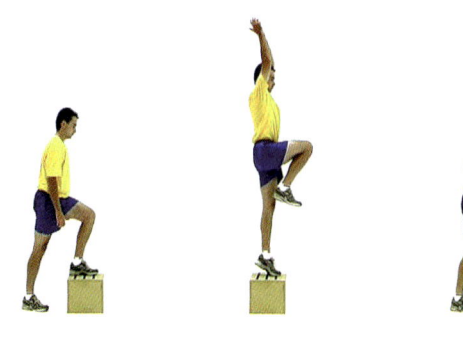

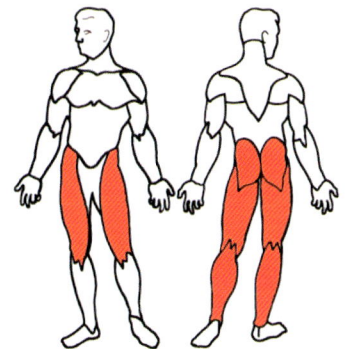

Single-leg front step-up.

81

CASE STUDIES: THE PRACTICAL APPLICATION OF CORE CONDITIONING

STRAIGHT LEG/ROMANIAN DEAD LIFT

4 x 8 repetitions. 30–45 seconds rest in between each set.
Speed of movement: 4-1-2 (count of 4 down, 1 when done, then 2 on return phase).

- Assume a parallel stance with the hands wide on the barbell.
- Begin with the bar close to the shins with the arms straight and the shoulders over the bar.
- Keep the chest up and look forward or slightly up with neutral curves in the spine.
- Flex at the hips until the bar travels below the knees then extend the hips to reverse the movement back to the start position.
- Complete the prescribed number of sets and repetitions.

Caution: do not flex the spine or allow the shoulders to round. Do not allow the hips to rise before the shoulders.

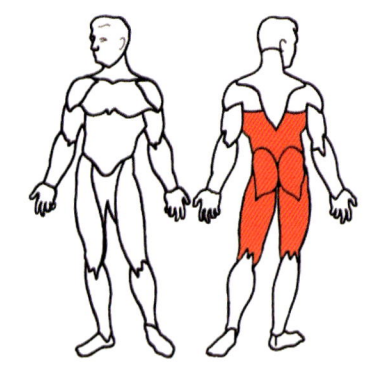

Single-leg lateral step-up.

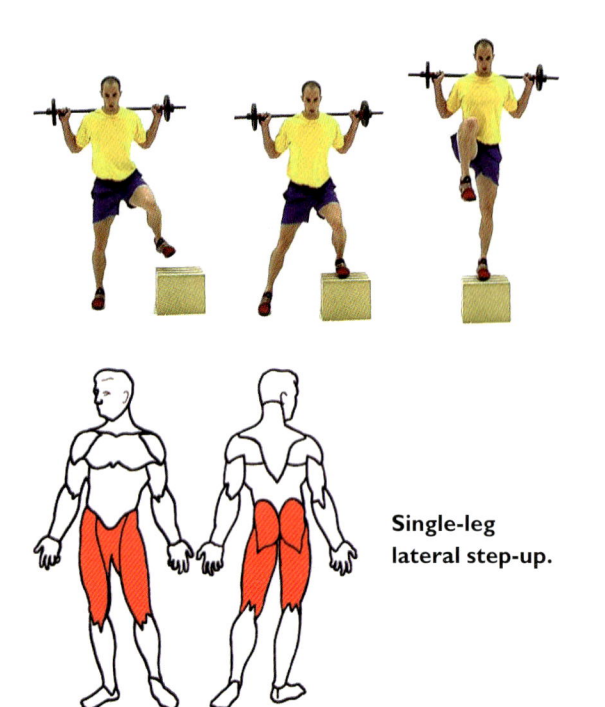

- Once you can increase the load, make sure that you place the barbell on your shoulders or hold the dumbbells by your side.
- Step straight on to the box with the working leg.
- Follow through with the other leg, raising the knee, to work your hip flexors.
- Lower back to the starting position.
- Complete the prescribed number of repetitions with one leg, and then switch legs.

Caution: ensure that the box is stable and do not allow the knees to buckle in. Keep tall and strong throughout the movement

Straight leg/ Romanian dead lift.

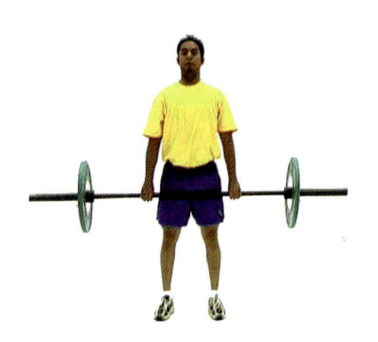

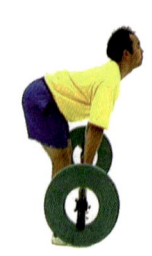

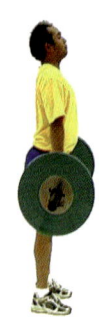

CASE STUDIES: THE PRACTICAL APPLICATION OF CORE CONDITIONING

STEP-DOWN STABILIZATION
3 x 8 left and right side.
Work alternate leg.

- Complete with body weight to begin with, then progress to loaded: secure the barbell on the upper trapezius muscles and not on the joints in the neck.
- Step forward off the box and balance on the one leg during the landing.
- Hold for 3 seconds and control the movement. This encourages a co-contraction of the quadriceps and hamstring muscles.
- The foot strike should be with the ball of the foot first.
- Allow the ankle, knee and hip to flex during the landing; the shoulders should be positioned above the knee with the leg directly under the hip.
- The box height should be around 30cm.
- Return to the box and complete the prescribed number of sets and repetition per leg.

Caution: the box should be sturdy and stable with a non-slip surface. Maintain a rigid torso and do not allow the torso to flex or collapse during contact with the ground. Maintain good posture ('branding') on landing.

- Contract the pelvic floor and use the core, pelvis and glutes to control the landing phase.
- The knee should track in line with the centre of the foot.
- Warm up adequately before commencing this exercise.

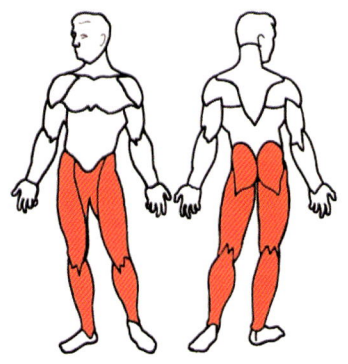

PLANK ARM-RAISE
3 x 8 left and right-side movement.
5 seconds rest in between each set.

- Start with the forearms flat on the ground and the elbows under the shoulders.
- Lift the knees off the floor, maintaining neutral curves in the spine and keeping the shoulder blades flat on the ribs.

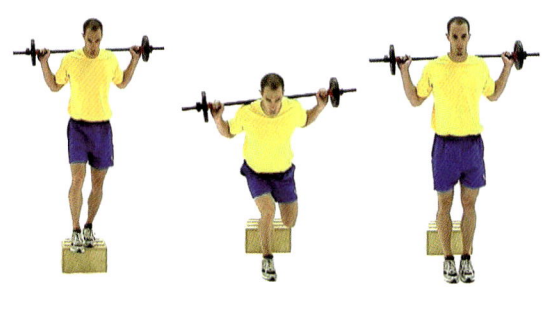

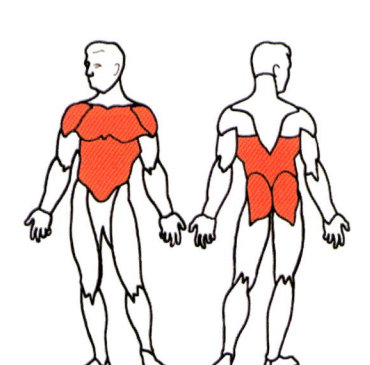

Step-down stabilization.

Plank arm-raise.

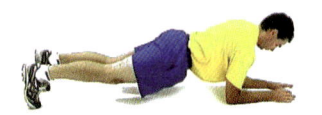

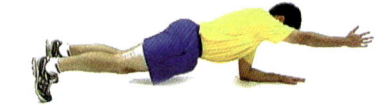

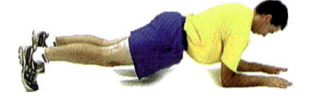

CASE STUDIES: THE PRACTICAL APPLICATION OF CORE CONDITIONING

- Take one arm off the floor and flex the shoulder while keeping the shoulders square.
- Keep the neck in line with the spine and try not to rotate the torso for this exercise.

Caution: do not allow the lower back to sag or the shoulder blades to wing or lift off the ribs.

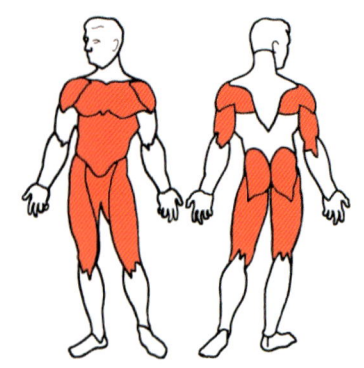

DUMBBELL LATERAL PULLOVER (ON FOAM ROLLER)

Dumbbell lateral pullover (on foam roller).

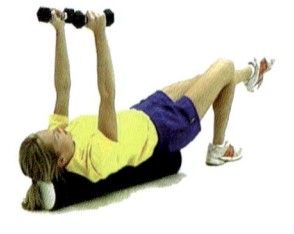

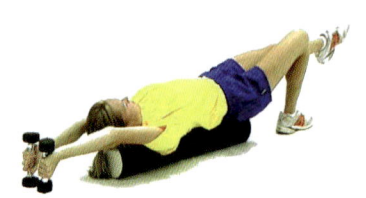

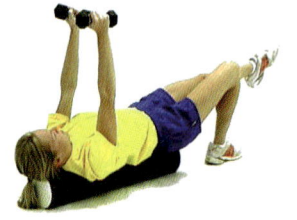

3 x 10 repetitions. Hold each rep for 3 seconds when extended, then return back to the start. Raise a leg on each repetition.
Use your breathing to stabilize.
Activate your pelvic floor.

- Ensure that the head and hips are supported on the roller with the foot flat on the ground.
- Keeping the arms parallel, lower the dumbbells until the hands are approximately in line with the shoulders.
- Then reverse the movement back to the start position.
- Maintain a neutral grip on the dumbbells and do not rotate the shoulders as the arms are lowering.

Caution: try to keep the rest of the body stable during the exercise.

GLUTE-HAM RAISE

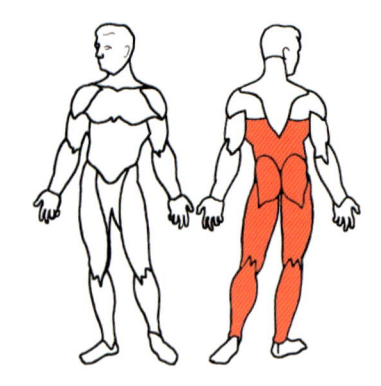

Glute-ham raise.

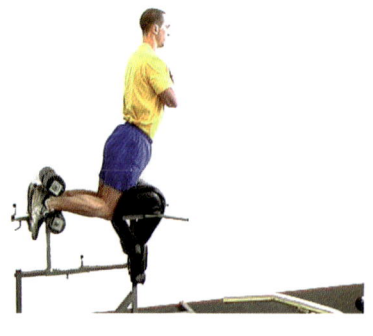

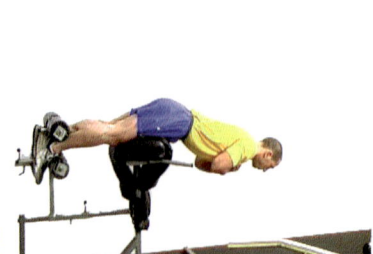

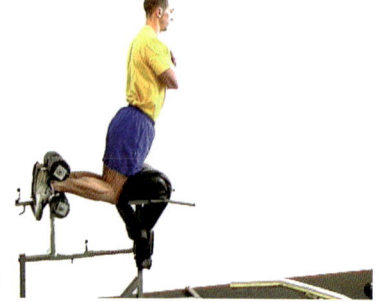

CASE STUDIES: THE PRACTICAL APPLICATION OF CORE CONDITIONING

4 sets x 8 repetitions.
30 seconds rest in between each set.

- Ensure that the feet are well supported and start with the knees on the pads.
- Place your arms over your chest and progress to holding a weight or place the hands behind the head to increase the difficulty.
- Keep the torso rigid.
- Maintaining a rigid torso, lower the torso at the knees until the shoulders are in line with or slightly below the level of the knees, then reverse the movements back to the start position.

Caution: warm up prior to commencing this exercise.

GOOD MORNING EXERCISE
4 sets x 8 repetitions.
30 seconds rest in between.

- Start with the bar resting behind the neck on the upper trapezius muscle.
- Lean forward at the hips with neutral curves in the spine until the torso is approximately parallel to the ground.
- While leaning forward, be sure to control the descent and keep the chest and chin up.
- At the end of the descent, extend to the starting position.

Caution: maintain the neutral curves in the spine through all phases of the exercises and do not round the shoulders. Keep the feet on the ground and control both phases of the lift. Look straight ahead or slightly up while leaning forward at the hips.

HAMSTRING HEEL FLICKS (STATIONARY)
Complete 3 sets of 20 repetitions left and right side. Work alternate sides.

- Start in an upright standing position.
- Work one leg at a time. Complete the functional movement pattern of hamstring flicks through a full range of movement as quickly as possible on the working limb.

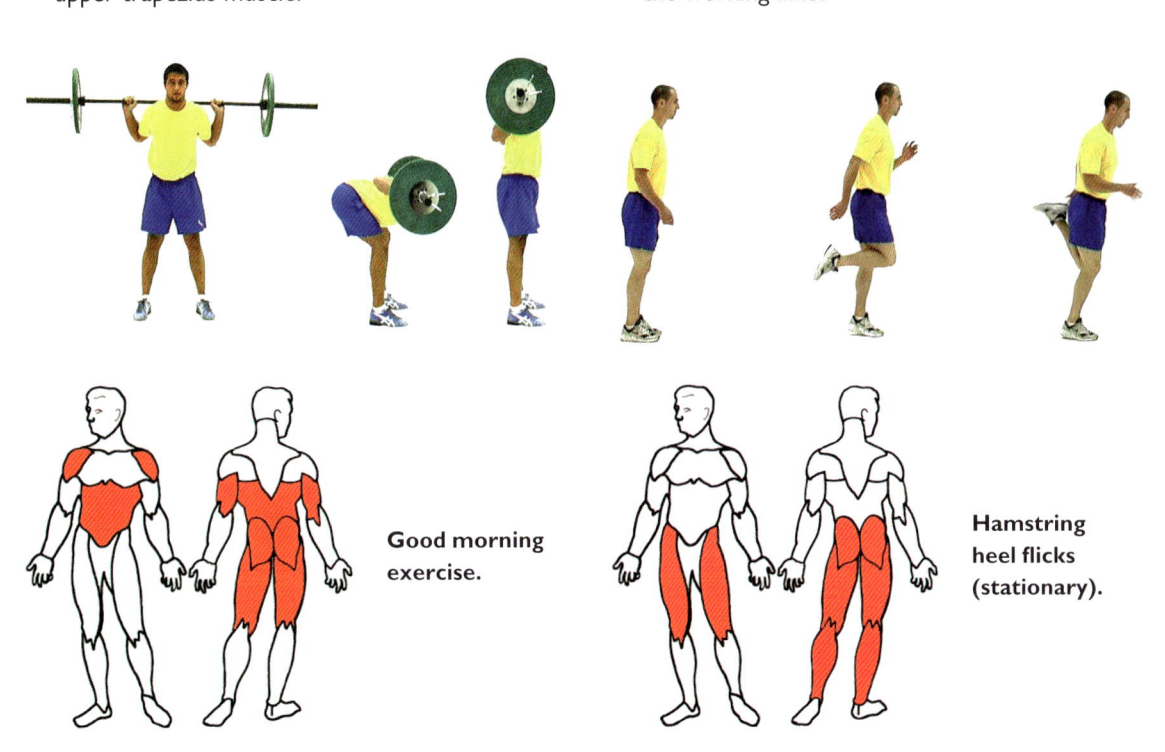

Good morning exercise.

Hamstring heel flicks (stationary).

- Stabilize on the standing leg. Think about posture, pelvic position and pelvic floor as you contact the hamstrings.
- Swap limbs after the prescribed duration.

Progressions

Exercises were progressed as follows:

- Increased load progression: worked to a repetition maximum. Many exercises were body weight to begin with, then progressed via external load (dumbbell/barbell).
- Client had good training history so knew how to push hard and place appropriate demands on her body and therefore progressed well.
- Decreased stability: exercises completed on BOSU/Swiss ball for example to increase challenge and body feedback/awareness.

Progressions of exercise selection:

- The long lever hip abduction progressed with the glute band and pulsing through range.
- Plank arm-raise progressed to leg lift, arm lift and to plank rotation.
- Single-leg bridging on the bench progressed to bridging on a Swiss ball for the added instability challenge and to demand more physical control.
- Romanian dead lift progressed with increased load, as did the good morning exercise.
- Other core exercises were added in, for example, seated oblique rotation with a medicine ball, alternating hip flexion/extension, kneeling arm-leg raise, Swiss ball roll-out stabilization. This was adjusted over the length of the programme to add variety and to keep the challenge as the client became more capable.

Outcome

- I saw the client on a weekly basis.
- Her commitment to make a positive change was very evident: she wants to run daily, it is very important to her and she would like to compete in 10k runs and even do another marathon if possible.
- Session RPE started at 3–5 (moderate–hard) and progressed to 5–8 (hard–very, very hard).
- Pain RPE was around 3 at the beginning of the plan with eccentric loading and normal running sessions. It reduced to zero–1 with running after 12 weeks of the plan.
- The client was educated about warm-up, mobility, myofascial release and slumps and completed a specific warm-up prior to any running-based activity. This was very helpful and ensured no pain when running.
- The client created a routine based upon the exercise prescription, which worked well for her pre-running preparation (see below).
- In addition to the warm-up guidelines I also provided a return-to-running plan for the client, to complement the strength and reconditioning plan. This 8-week bespoke plan took the client from 'rehab' runs to more functional progressions and then increased volume and intensity to target a 10k distance. This was achieved as prescribed.
- The client's attention to detail to provide herself with the best possible outcome was excellent and really made a difference for her. She worked hard and reaped the benefit.
- The client is aware that she needs to continue to keep her glutes and core strong and must continue with her eccentric loading for her hamstrings on a regular basis. With her adherence and resultant positive outcome, her goal of being able to run pain-free has been achieved.

Client's Pre-Running Routine:
Warm-Up and Dynamic Flex Exercises:
Completed prior to every run:

- Foam roll/myofascial release: calves, quads, hamstrings and glutes.

- Lumbar spine mobility.
- Slumps: 3 x 8 left and right side (alternate leg).
- Glute band activation: 3 x left and right side to fatigue.
- Good morning exercise: 3 x 8 repetitions, 10 seconds rest in between.
- 4–5 minutes of multi-directional movement patterns progressing from straight-line running, side slides, high knees, kick bum, backward running and turn, accelerations and gradually increase the intensity over time.

This warm-up is followed by some dynamic flexibility exercises. Stretches are held for only 2–3 seconds and each exercise/movement pattern is performed for up to 20–30 seconds:

- Hamstring heel flicks.
- Hamstring/leg extensions (push leg out towards the front of your body, return to start position, switch leg).
- Bent-over hamstrings (sweep the floor with your hands, leg out straight in front of you, toe pointing up).
- Quad stretch (good position, standing upright).
- Groin stretch (feet wide, move side to side, easing through the groins).
- Hip flexor stretch (in a lunge position, tilt your pelvis forwards and feel a stretch through the front of the back lunging leg. To increase the stretch, put the same arm in the air as the leg that is lunged backwards and reach up high).
- Straight-leg calf stretch and bent-knee calf stretch.

Continue with the multi-directional work for an additional 3–4 minutes, increasing in intensity. Include some progressive sprints and increased-intensity change-of-direction movements (forwards and backwards). Finish off with another dynamic stretch of whatever you need in preparation for activity.

Total duration approximately 15–20 minutes.

Bent-knee push backs: mini squat position then extend knees with flexed hips to really feel upper hamstring area: 3 x 8. 10 seconds rest in between. After each session: foam roll.

CASE STUDY 5

Assessment

Diagnosis: Post-partum diastasis recti, also known as recti divarication.

Definition:
It is common for the two muscles that run down the middle of the stomach to separate during pregnancy, because the growing womb (uterus) pushes them apart, making them longer and weaker. This is sometimes called diastasis recti, or recti divarication. The degree of separation varies from one woman to another. After birth, it can be assessed using this simple technique:

- Lie on your back with your legs bent and your feet flat on the floor.
- Raise your shoulders off the floor slightly and look down at your tummy.
- Using the tips of your fingers, feel between the edges of the muscles, above and below your belly button. See how many fingers you can fit into the gap between your muscles.
- Do this regularly to check that the gap is gradually decreasing.

The separation between the stomach muscles usually goes back to normal about eight weeks after the birth. If the gap is still obvious at eight weeks, the muscles may still be long and weak, which can increase the risk of low back problems (https://www.nhs.uk/Conditions/pregnancy-and-baby/Pages/your-body-after-childbirth.aspx).

Current presentation:
12 weeks after delivery. Generally tired but as to be expected with second baby. Working on pelvic floor control and has been throughout pregnancy. Natural

CASE STUDIES: THE PRACTICAL APPLICATION OF CORE CONDITIONING

Needs Analysis

Client name	Client # 5
Occupation	Self-employed
DOB/age	35 years old
Sports/physical activities completed	Running, tennis, hockey – general fitness.
Training history	Have exercised all my life, enjoy the physical side and also the social side of things.
Injury history Please Include date of injury, surgical dates, investigations/scans, left/right side, etc. Please be as specific as possible.	Second pregnancy. Everything went well, natural labour (same for baby #1) but have been diagnosed with diastasis recti 8 weeks after delivery. The gap between my abdominals is quite wide and I have been told that I need to improve my core strength to help it reduce back to normal. Had low back pain the last few weeks of both pregnancies, which was quite limiting.
Goals/training targets e.g. stronger legs, leaner, general fitness improvement, upcoming events and dates	Reduce gap in abdominals. Gain strength after pregnancies to help reduce back pain. Return to hockey, tennis, etc.
Commitments e.g. work, family, time constraints, etc.	Full-time mother.
Gym access and facilities	I am a member of a gym and have some home-based gym equipment as well: Swiss ball, mat, and dumbbells.
Referring practitioner (if relevant)	GP and midwife.
Any other relevant information	Everything else uncomplicated in pregnancy. Feel good. Generally tired but normal with a new baby and also baby #1 needing things! Breast-feeding.

labour for both children. The diastasis distance between the client's rectus abdominis was measured as 4cm on average over three measurement sites: belly button, midline and base of abdominals.

Exercise prescription:

- Prescribed session to be completed 2–3 x each day for first 6–8 weeks.
- Completed daily.
- The client saw me every week for contact time and appropriate progressions.
- Good body awareness and control were essential.

Other things to consider:
Targets:

- Improve control and activation.
- Use breathing and bracing during exercises.
- Reduce diastasis distance and improve strength.

CASE STUDIES: THE PRACTICAL APPLICATION OF CORE CONDITIONING

Challenges/concerns:

- Fatigue: the client was tired with a new baby, breast-feeding and looking after her toddler!

Strength and Conditioning Plan

Checklist:

- Isometric contractions, breathing, bracing and control coached and encouraged.
- Ensure excellent body awareness throughout and regular pelvic floor work.
- Session was with baby and completed in a relaxed manner.

Frequency:

- Strength programme to be completed 2–3 × each day for the first 6–8 weeks.

Session duration:

Session took between 10–15 minutes.
When I saw the client, I reviewed all of the prescribed exercises to ensure excellent technique and understanding.

Intensity:

Borg Rating of Perceived Exertion (RPE) = 2–3 (easy–moderate) to begin with, to establish confidence and a sense of movement/feeling in and around abdominals.
Target pain scale: zero. No pain in abdominals. Still experiencing intermittent low back pain.

Note to client:

- All exercises should be completed with absolute attention to detail and with excellent technique.
- Modify how you lift the children: brace as you lift.
- Also activate your pelvic floor as you lift and move.
- Activate pelvic floor muscles as you complete the exercises and throughout the day.
- Work on your body awareness and know where you should feel the muscles work.

Core-Strengthening Session:

- Warm-up/activation before every session (see Pelvic Tilt, below).
- Then continue with the options below.
- Complete 3–4 of the 8 options 2–3 × each day.
- Vary which option you select.

PELVIC FLOOR EXERCISES

Pelvic floor exercises strengthen the muscles around the bladder, vagina or penis, and back passage. Strengthening the pelvic floor muscles can help stop incontinence, treat prolapse, and make sex better, too. Both men and women can benefit. The pelvic floor muscles may be identified by trying to stop the flow of urine midstream, however, doing this regularly is not recommended, as it can be harmful to the bladder.

To strengthen your pelvic floor muscles, sit comfortably and squeeze the muscles 10–15 times in a row. Do not hold your breath or tighten your stomach, buttock or thigh muscles at the same time. When you get used to doing pelvic floor exercises, you can try holding each squeeze for a few seconds. Every week, you can add more squeezes, but be careful not to overdo it and always have a rest between sets of squeezes. After a few months, you should start to notice the results, but you should still carry on doing the exercises. If you are pregnant or planning to get pregnant, it is wise to start doing pelvic floor exercises straight away. Having a strong pelvic floor will lower the risk of incontinence after the birth, and can also help with delivery.

CASE STUDIES: THE PRACTICAL APPLICATION OF CORE CONDITIONING

- Focus on control, activation and breathing on every exercise.

PELVIC TILT

- Lie on your back with your knees bent and a pillow under your hips and another pillow between your knees.
- Feet flat on the floor and your arms at your sides or placed on your abdominals for feedback.
- Inhale, then exhale and draw your abdominals in, imagine your belly button moving towards your spine and brace your abdominal muscles at the same time.
- Tuck your pelvis under slightly (posterior tilt) and squeeze your glutes as you contract your pelvic floor muscles.
- Hold 5 seconds and release. Complete 10 repetitions.

DOUBLE-LEG BRIDGING (WITH BAND AROUND KNEES)

3 x 6–8 repetitions.
Hold each raise/rep for 3–4 seconds.
Use your breathing. Pull your belly button towards your spine and big belly breath out, as if blowing away a ping pong ball, and brace.

Progression: feet on to bench:

- Start with the feet approximately shoulder width apart with the head and shoulders in contact with the ground.
- Lift the hips off the ground until the thighs are in line with the torso.
- Hold for 3–4 seconds, and then control the movement back to the start position, feeling each vertebra return to the starting position.

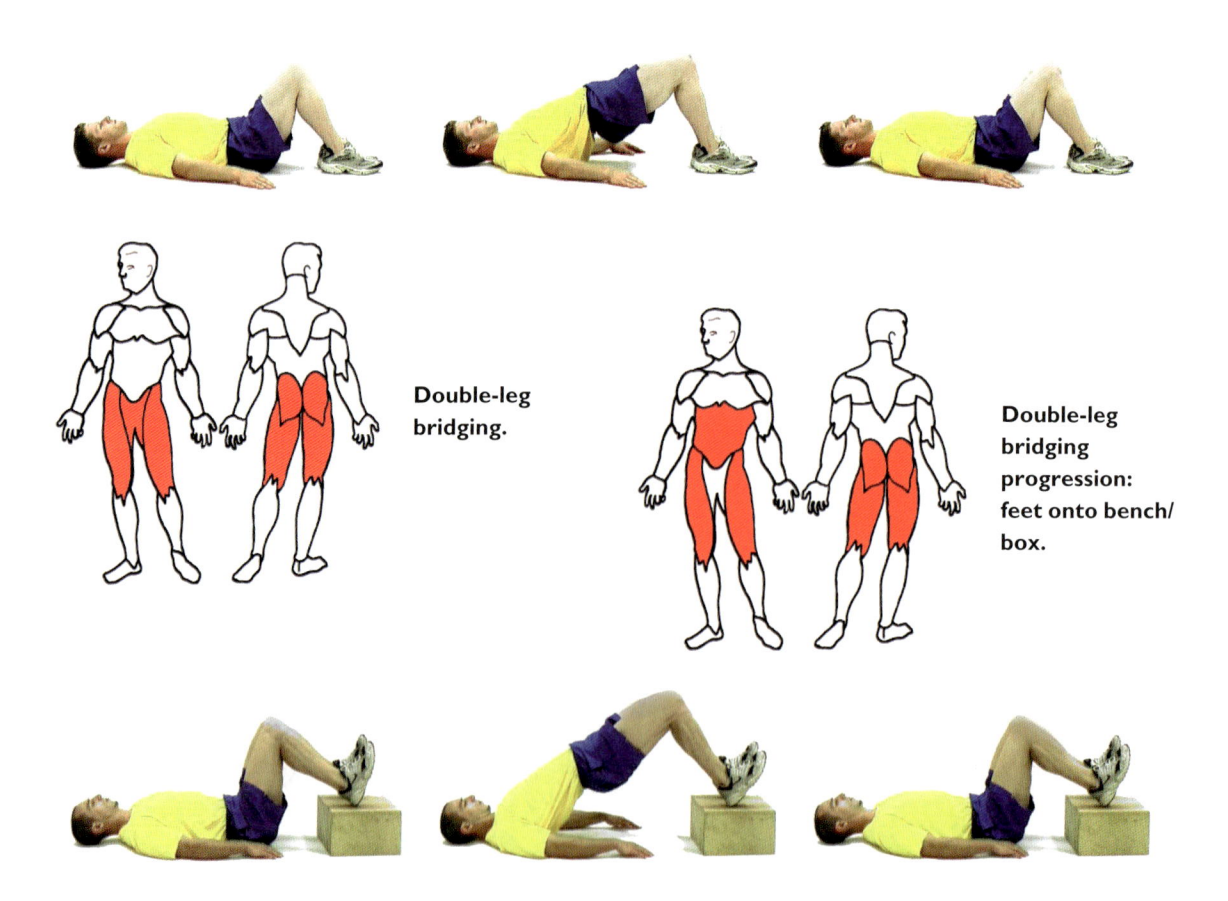

Double-leg bridging.

Double-leg bridging progression: feet onto bench/box.

CASE STUDIES: THE PRACTICAL APPLICATION OF CORE CONDITIONING

- Complete the prescribed number of sets and repetitions.
- Do not forget to breathe throughout the exercise: don't hold your breath.

KNEELING ARM-LEG RAISE

Brace in this prone position so sensation of abdominal wall falling away is avoided.
3 x 10 L and R (20 total alternate reps).
20 seconds rest in between sets.

- Start with the hands under the shoulders, the knees under the hips and neutral curves in the spine.
- Extend the hip and knee and extend the opposite shoulder.
- Hold for 3 seconds then return back to the four-point kneeling position.

- Repeat the movements with both limbs in an alternating fashion for the prescribed number of sets and repetitions.

Caution: Do not allow the spine to round or sag, especially as you get fatigued. Brace through the abdominals whilst in this prone position.

HIP FLEXION ABDUCTION

2 x sets of 6–8 left and right side.
Work alternate sides.

- The head, shoulders and hips should remain on the floor.
- Flex and abduct the hip to lower the leg towards the ground then return the thigh to the start position.

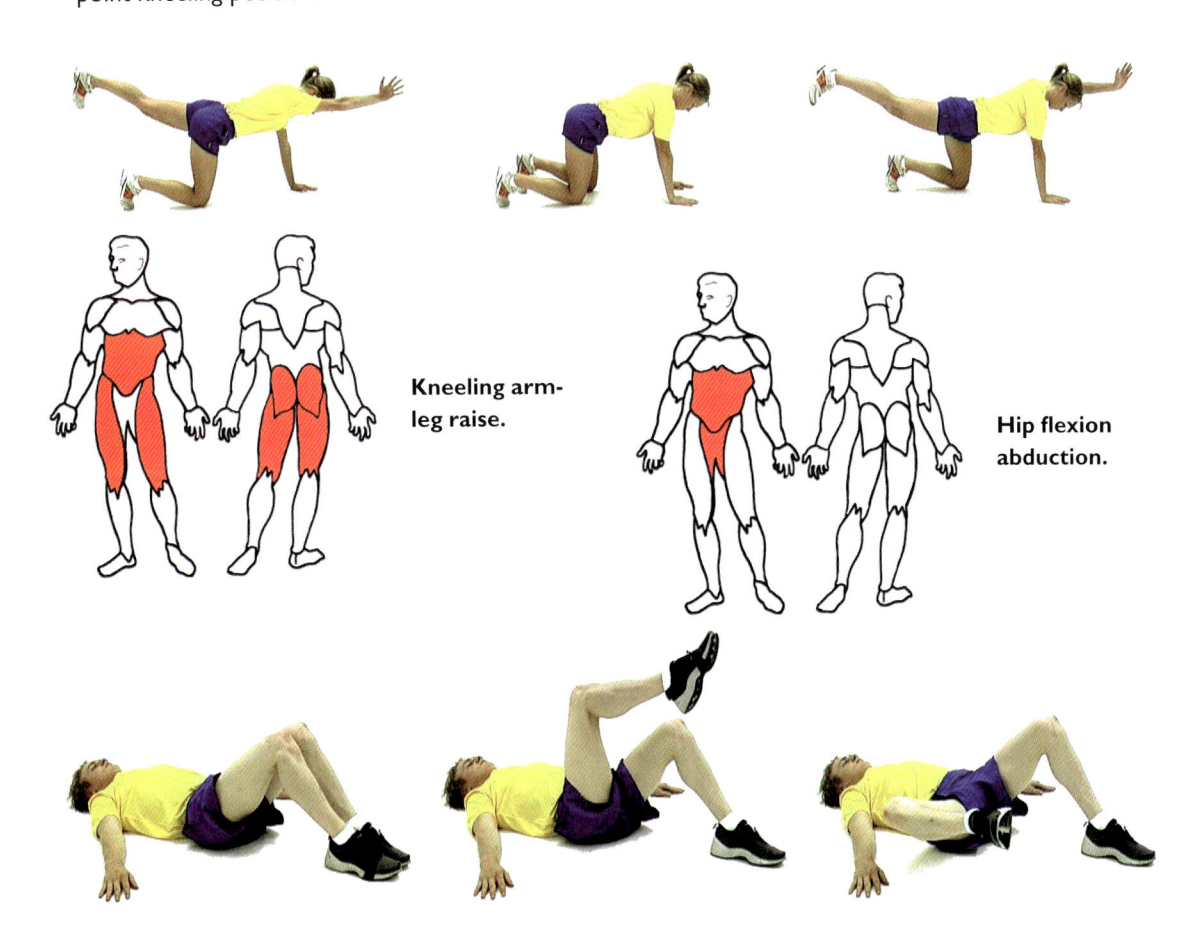

Kneeling arm-leg raise.

Hip flexion abduction.

CASE STUDIES: THE PRACTICAL APPLICATION OF CORE CONDITIONING

- Keep the pelvis stable and in a neutral position throughout the exercise.
- Draw the belly button in before abducting the hip.

Caution: do not extend the neck or the spine during the exercise.

BOX BRIDGING WITH ISOMETRIC BALL HOLDS (CAN ALSO BE COMPLETED WITH A SWISS BALL)

3 x 8 holds.
Place a ball or medicine ball between your knees.
Squeeze the ball and hold for 3–4 seconds during upward hold phase.
Belly breath out as you brace, lift, squeeze and hold.
10 seconds rest in between each set.

- Position the feet securely on the bench with the hands on the floor.
- The knees should be flexed to around 90 degrees and a ball placed in between the knees.
- Lift the hips off the floor until the legs are in line with the torso, and hold as directed.
- Reverse the movement back to the start position.
- Vary the position of the hands on the floor to assist with balance.
- Place the hands across the chest to progress the exercise.

Caution: do not raise the body too high off the floor.

FOUR-POINT STABILIZATION

Work for duration: build up from 10-second holds to 30-second holds.

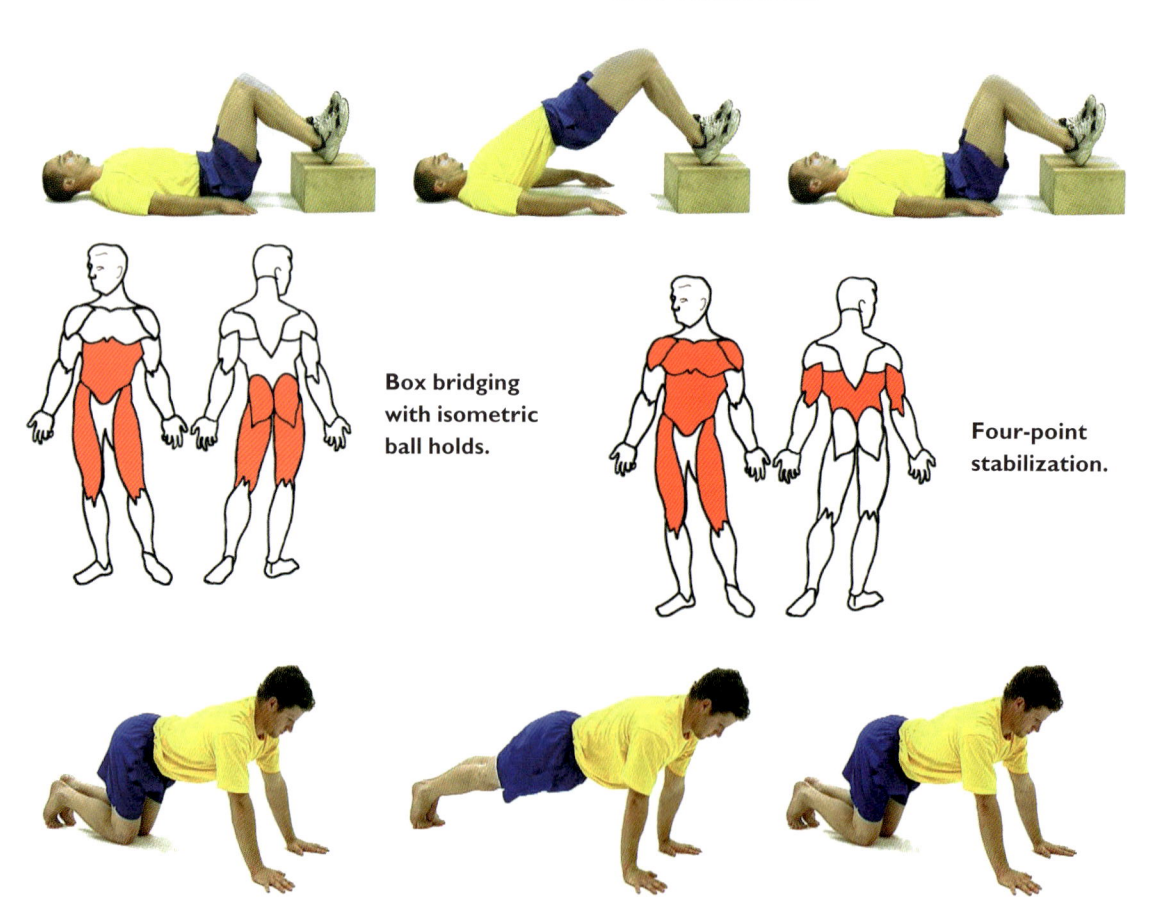

Box bridging with isometric ball holds.

Four-point stabilization.

CASE STUDIES: THE PRACTICAL APPLICATION OF CORE CONDITIONING

Complete 3–4 sets.
5 seconds rest in between each set.

- Assume a front support position with the hands underneath the shoulders and neutral curves of the spine.
- Extend the hips and knees to press up to a front support position while keeping the torso rigid.
- Draw the belly button in and brace before lifting upwards.
- Hold for the prescribed duration then reverse the movements back to the start position.
- Control both phases of the exercise, particularly the lowering phase.
- Consider placing a mat under the hands for additional comfort.

Caution: keep the neck in line with the spine and do not allow the spine to sag.

THE CLAM
3 sets left and right side to fatigue (feel the burn!)

- Perform this exercise without a band to begin with (unlike in the image).
- Progress to a band when you require more resistance to get the same feeling of fatigue.
- Side lie on the floor and bend your knees together
- Relax your upper body and activate your core: pull your belly button towards your spine.
- Start with the hips and shoulders square then externally rotate the hip (lift it off the other knee like a clam).
- Try to keep the rest of the body stationary as the hip rotates.

- Return to the start position and repeat for the prescribed number of sets and repetitions in a slow and controlled manner.

SUPINE SWISS BALL BRIDGING WITH HIP FLEXION
Initially start with just holding the position for 10–30 seconds.
Contract your pelvic floor muscles and brace through your spine. Breathe as you hold this position.

- Start with the head and shoulders on the stability ball with the knees in line with the hips and the feet under the knees.
- Hold each raise/rep for 3–4 seconds. Belly breathe and control as you lift.
- Do not allow your belly to bulge as you lift a leg. Pull/draw your belly button towards your spine and place the hands across your abdominals to ensure no bulging and good position.
- Progress to including a leg lift within the 30-second hold. Alternate left and right leg lifts with excellent control.
- When strength and control improve, progress to 3 x 6–10 repetitions L and R as you maintain the position.

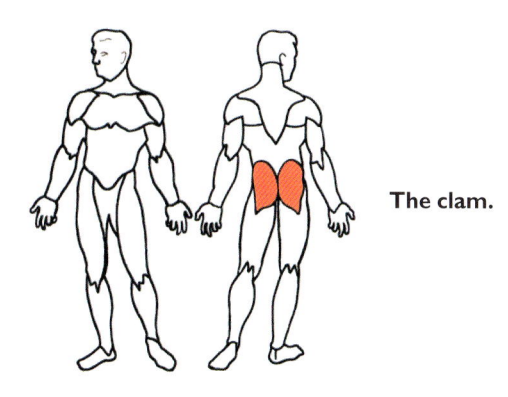

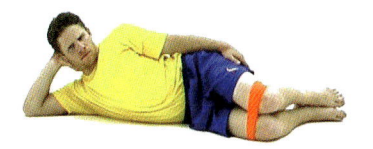

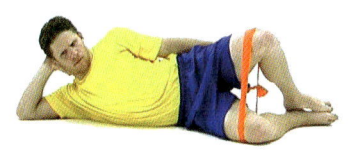

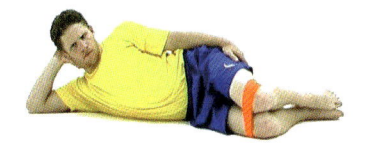

The clam.

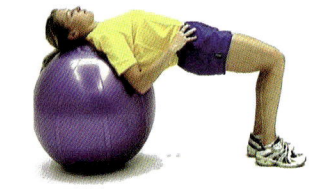

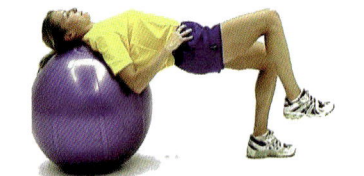

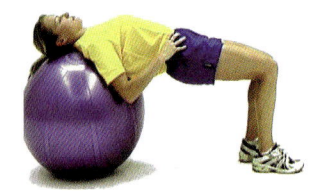

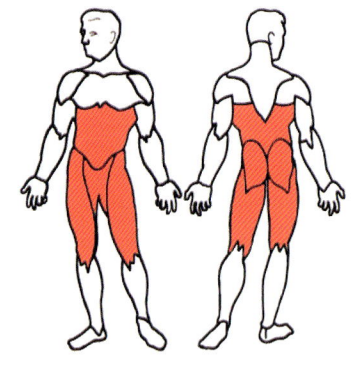

CASE STUDIES: THE PRACTICAL APPLICATION OF CORE CONDITIONING

Supine Swiss ball bridging with hip flexion.

- Repeat the movements with the same leg or alternate the legs continuously.

Caution: maintain a neutral and level pelvic position and do not allow the lower back to excessively extend.

KNEELING CABLE PUSH PRESS AND ROTATION VARIATIONS

Work for duration: build up from 10 second holds to 30 second holds.
Complete 3–4 sets.

- Consider placing a mat or towel under the knee and hold both ends of the rope.
- Changing the leg that is forward alters the emphasis on the abdominal muscles and should be done through intermittent periods during the exercise.
- Maintaining an erect torso position, pull the cable down and across the body in a diagonal pattern, a forward push position (isometric hold) and work for the prescribed duration.
- Contract your pelvic floor, brace and pull your belly button towards your spine.
- Belly breathe throughout in a 'strong, braced' position.

Caution: maintain a firm grip on the rope. Change the position where you hold the rope to vary the load through the abdominals.

No supplementary exercises were required at this point, but the client was keen to start more

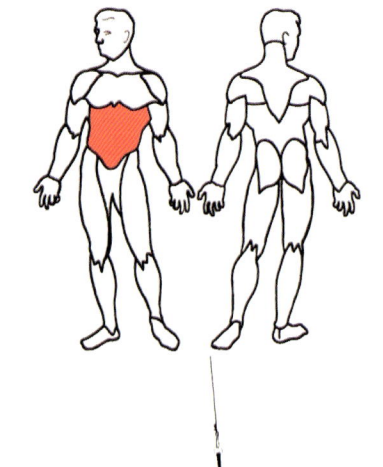

Kneeling cable push press.

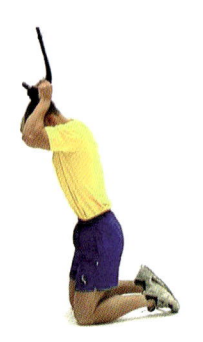

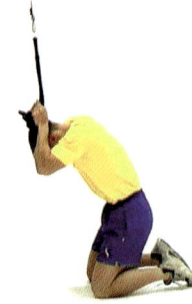

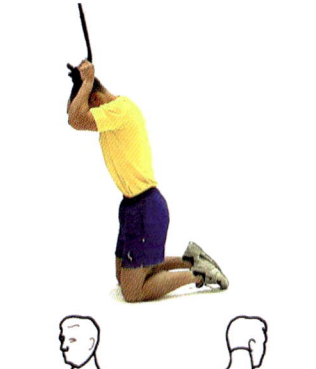

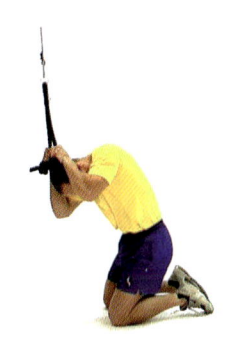

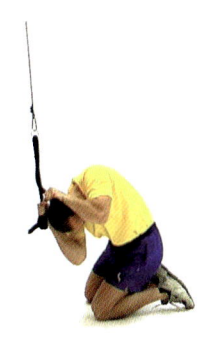

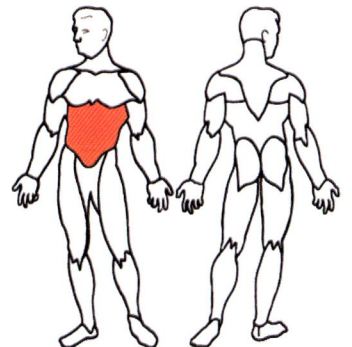

CASE STUDIES: THE PRACTICAL APPLICATION OF CORE CONDITIONING

Kneeling cable rotation.

functional exercises once she had addressed the development of her core strength.

Progressions

Exercises were progressed as follows:

- Increased movement: from isometric holds to gradual movement, with a focus on maintaining a brace position, pulling the belly button towards the spine and no abdominal bulge. Ensure excellent control.
- Progressions included increased repetitions or duration as well as decreased stability, for example, progressing to kneeling on a BOSU or seated on a Swiss ball on the cable push press and rotation.

Progressions of exercise selection:

- Activities began in an isometric-based phase, slow and controlled, to establish confidence, good activation, control and understanding.
- Every exercise was progressed: light 1kg dumbbells held on the kneeling arm-leg raise, increased load on the cable work, leg lift introduced on the supine Swiss ball bridging, pulsing progression with the clam and also an introduction of the long lever abduction with a band as well.

Outcome

- I saw the client on average every week to two weeks.
- Her commitment and adherence to the programme were very good, generally completing at least 2 sessions of 10–15 minutes every day. On most days the client completed all three daily sessions.
- This was achievable as she was based at home with the new baby every day, so the plan was easily slotted into her daily routine.
- Fatigue (lack of sleep due to new baby) was the main cause of non-compliance, but this was rare.
- The client was nervous to begin with, knowing that she had a reasonably significant diastasis, but her progress was good.
- Session RPE progressed over the weeks from 2–3 (easy–moderate) to around RPE 5–6 (hard) and after the first few weeks of creating confidence and exercise familiarity, the client was able to work at a good intensity.
- The client's low back pain reduced and completely disappeared by around week 6 of the plan, and her diastasis recti was beginning to reduce in size.

CASE STUDIES: THE PRACTICAL APPLICATION OF CORE CONDITIONING

- The client was in touch with her midwife and also had intermittent appointments with her GP to see how the diastasis recti was reducing. She was advised that it may take between 3 months to a year to reduce, but signs were good. Her clinical presentation of low back pain had gone as a result of developing a stronger core, and achieving better postural and pelvic control and a stronger posterior chain.
- We discussed that this is a long-term commitment to core strength and stability. As the client has an active background, this is something that she is committed to include in her training on a regular basis.

CASE STUDY 6

Assessment

Diagnosis: Adductor/groin strain: Grade II.

Definition:
A groin strain is a tear or rupture to any one of the adductor muscles, resulting in pain in the inner thigh. Groin injuries can range from very mild to

DEFINITIONS OF GRADES OF MUSCULAR INJURY

Grade I Muscle Strain

There is damage to individual muscle fibres (less than 5 per cent of fibres). This is a mild strain that requires 2 to 3 weeks' rest.

Grade II Muscle Strain

There is more extensive damage, with more muscle fibres involved, but the muscle is not completely ruptured. The rest period required is usually between 3 and 6 weeks.

Grade III Muscle Strain

There is a complete rupture of a muscle. In a sports person this will usually require surgery to repair the muscle. The rehabilitation time is around 3 months.
(www.physioroom.com)

Needs Analysis

Client name	Client # 6
Occupation	Graduate
DOB/age	22 years old
Sports/physical activities completed	Football player: trains 2 x each week with a game on the weekend. Plays in the midfield.
Training history	Played all kinds of sports through school and university. Keen sportsman: rugby, cricket, football, badminton. Also go to the gym to lift weights and train.
Injury history *Please Include date of injury, surgical dates, investigations/scans, left/right side, etc. Please be as specific as possible.*	Playing football 70 minutes into the game slid into a tackle and over-reached. I felt a sharp pain in my left groin area. I came off and iced the area. Have been seeing a chartered physiotherapist for 5 weeks. They recommended seeing you now that the area is starting to heal.

CASE STUDIES: THE PRACTICAL APPLICATION OF CORE CONDITIONING

Goals/training targets *e.g. stronger legs, leaner, general fitness improvement, upcoming events and dates*	Rehab fully from groin strain. Become stronger. Reduce risk of re-injury.
Commitments *e.g. work, family, time constraints, etc.*	Graduate student. Recently out of university. Gap year/looking for work.
Gym access and facilities	I am a member of a gym.
Referring practitioner (if relevant)	Chartered Physiotherapist
Any other relevant information	Will work hard. Want to get back to training and football ready for pre-season.

very severe and completely debilitating. The main symptom of an acute groin strain is a sudden sharp pain in the groin area, either in the belly of the muscle or higher up where the tendon attaches to the pelvic bone. It might be felt when sprinting or changing direction quickly. The athlete may or may not be able to play on, depending on the severity of the injury (http://www.sportsinjuryclinic.net/sport-injuries/hip-groin-pain/groin-strain).

Current presentation:
Clinically quiet. Physiotherapist is very happy with progress and feels that the client is ready to progress his rehabilitation and conditioning.

Exercise prescription:

- Strength/reconditioning programme to be completed 3 x each week.
- Hip mobility session.

Other things to consider:
Targets:

- Close contact/liaison with physiotherapist for rehab and exercise prescription. Good multidisciplinary work to benefit the client.
- Consider overall conditioning for the client to ensure that when he returns to football he is well conditioned in all other components of fitness, therefore prescribe off-feet conditioning, pool work, strength work, core conditioning and specific rehabilitation to be planned within the programme.

Challenges/concerns:

- Improve body awareness of the client: it is his first injury and he is eager to get back as soon as possible.
- Discussed long-term gain of becoming stronger and that my philosophy is that he will return as a better athlete as a result of the injury.
- Gradual loading: again ensuring that the client understands the progressive overload and attention to detail with movement patterns.

Strength and Conditioning Plan

Checklist:
Rehabilitation and reconditioning programme prescribed to address the following:

- Groin/adductor specific rehabilitation.
- Football-specific conditioning to include off-feet and progressive return to play plan in addition to complementary strength and conditioning plan.

CASE STUDIES: THE PRACTICAL APPLICATION OF CORE CONDITIONING

Frequency:

- Hip mobility/warm-up to be completed before any physical work.
- Strength and conditioning programme to be completed 3 x each week.

Session duration:
Session took 60 minutes to complete plus cardio-vascular/interval sessions.

Intensity:
Borg Rating of Perceived Exertion (RPE) = 2–3 (easy–moderate) to begin with, then progressed to full intensity with an RPE of 8–10 (very, very hard–maximal) in line with the demands of the game.

Target pain scale: 1 or zero. Experiences some intermittent dull aching on the injury site. Still has 3–4 sessions with the physiotherapist planned.

Note to client:

- All exercises should be completed with absolute attention to detail and with excellent technique.
- Improve body awareness and prepare mentally for a good rehab phase (being injured is a new thing for this client).
- Recognize that if you stick with the plan you will be more robust and a better athlete as a result.
- Work on your body awareness and know where you should feel the muscles work.
- Report any pain, irritation or problems as soon as possible.

HIP/GROIN MOBILITY SESSION

To be completed prior to every conditioning session:

- 2 x 20–30 seconds on each exercise L and R side.
- Select 5–6 exercises out of the 10 options.
- Vary your selection.
- Hip/groin mobility should take around 10 minutes when familiar with the exercises and should become part of your pre-match/training preparation routine.

HIP ROTATION ('CLOSE THE GATE')

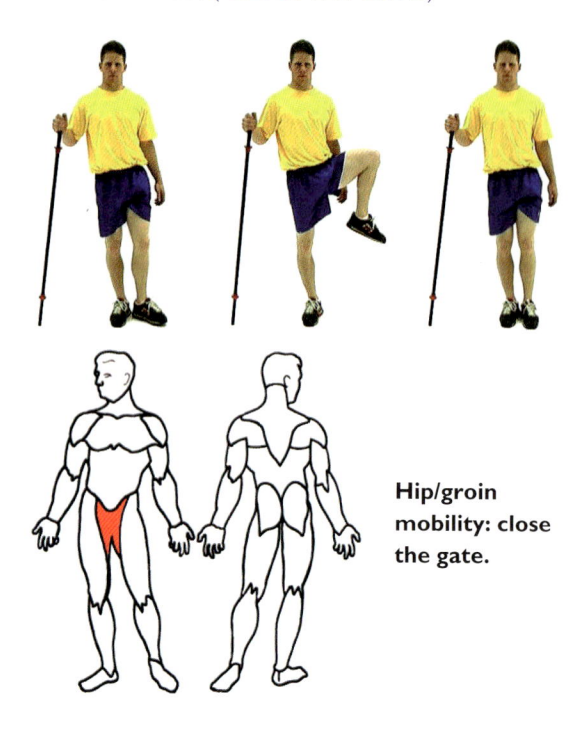

Hip/groin mobility: close the gate.

- Simultaneously abduct and flex the hip to approximately 90 degrees, then horizontally adduct the hip.
- Gradually increase the range as the mobility of the hip improves.
- The movements should begin smooth and the speed should be gradually increased if necessary.

Caution: the movements should be at the hips and not the spine. Discontinue the stretch if pain or discomfort is experienced in the hip joint.

HIP ROTATION ('OPEN THE GATE')

- Flex the hip to approximately 90 degrees, horizontally abduct the hip and then return the foot to the start position.
- Try to keep the hips and shoulders facing forward during the movements.
- Gradually increase the range as the mobility of the hip improves.
- The movements should begin smooth and gradually increase the speed if necessary.

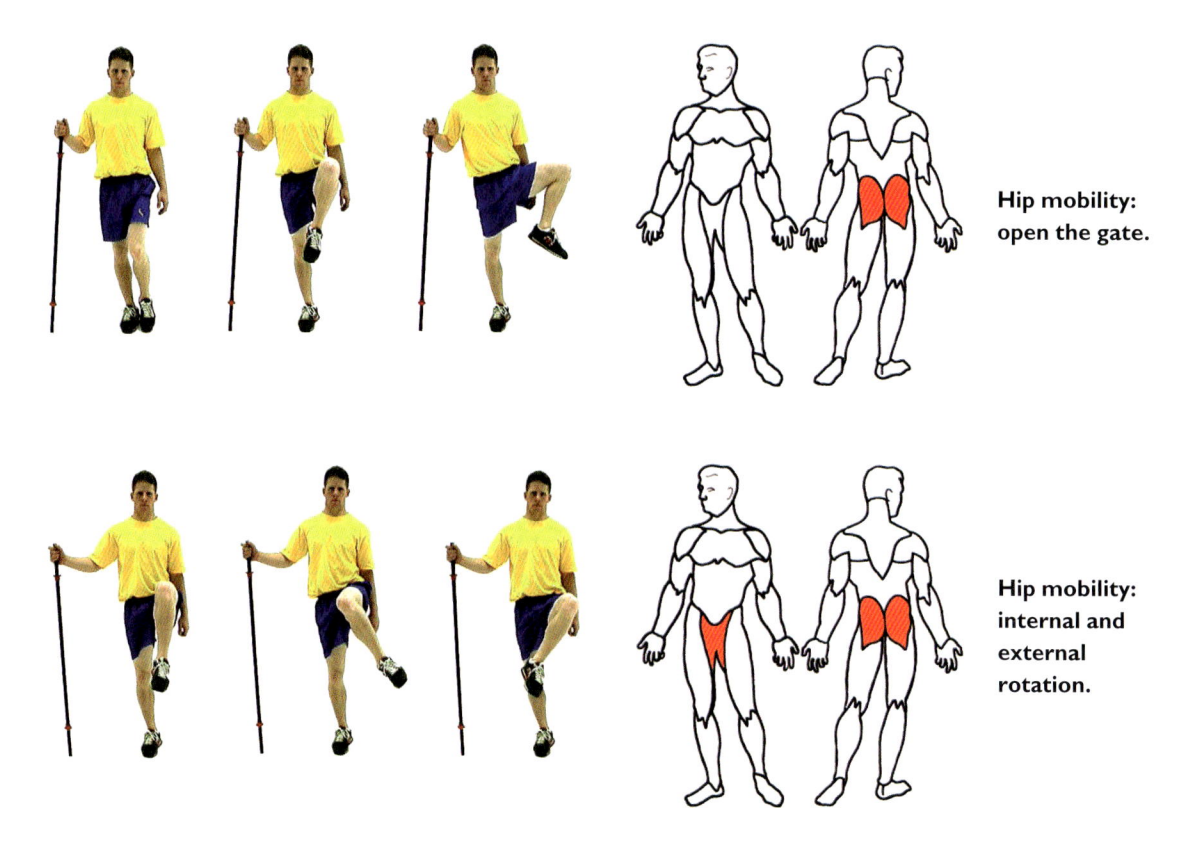

CASE STUDIES: THE PRACTICAL APPLICATION OF CORE CONDITIONING

Hip mobility: open the gate.

Hip mobility: internal and external rotation.

Caution: the movements should be at the hips and not the spine. Discontinue the stretch if pain or discomfort is experienced in the hip joint.

HIP ROTATION: INTERNAL AND EXTERNAL ROTATION

3 x 8 repetitions (internal and external movement = 1 rep).
Work alternate leg.

- Start with the hip flexed to approximately 90 degrees.
- Maintaining the same horizontal position of the thigh, internally and externally rotate the hip.
- Gradually increase the range as the mobility of the hip improves.

Caution: the movements should be at the hips and not the spine. Discontinue the stretch if pain or discomfort is experienced in the hip joint.

SIDE-LYING HIP EXTENSION – FLEXION

3 x 8 left and right side.
Work alternate sides.

- Keep the neck in line with the spine and the bottom elbow under the shoulder.
- Lift the top leg and flex and extend the hip, keeping the upper body stationary.
- The range of movement may vary depending on the requirements of the exercise.
- Place a weight cuff around the ankle to increase the resistance for this exercise over time.

Caution: maintain a rigid torso and do not rotate it during the movement.

HIP FLEXION ABDUCTION

2 x 6–8 left and right side.
Work alternate leg.

CASE STUDIES: THE PRACTICAL APPLICATION OF CORE CONDITIONING

Side-lying hip extension – flexion.

Hip flexion abduction.

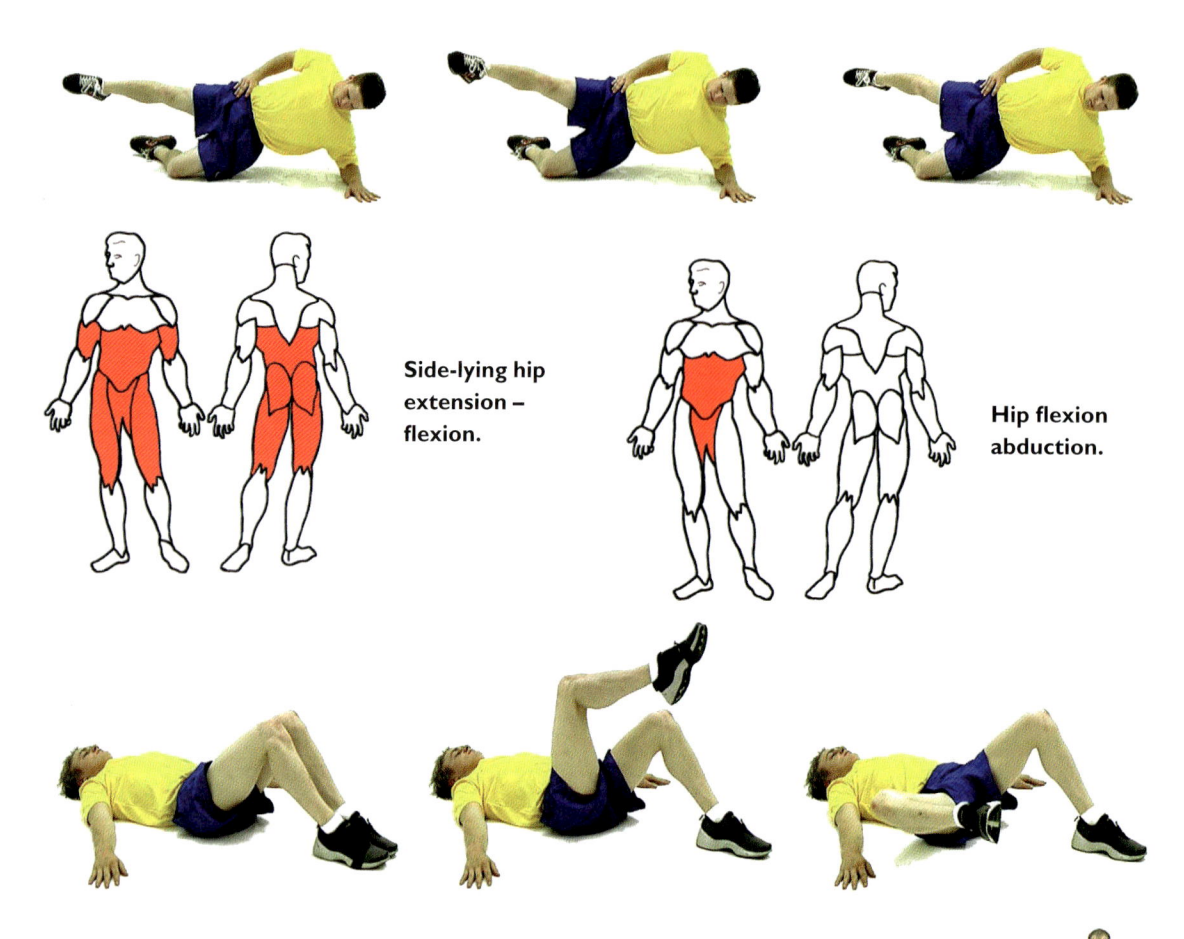

- The head, shoulders and hips should remain on the floor.
- Flex and abduct the hip to lower the leg towards the ground, then return the thigh to the start position.
- Keep the pelvis stable and in a neutral position throughout the exercise.

Caution: do not extend the neck or the spine during the exercise.

LATERAL LUNGE HIP FLEXION
2 x 8 left and right side.
Use cones/hurdle for movement patterning.

- Lunge to the side in a low position then extend and flex the hip while continuing to move sideways.

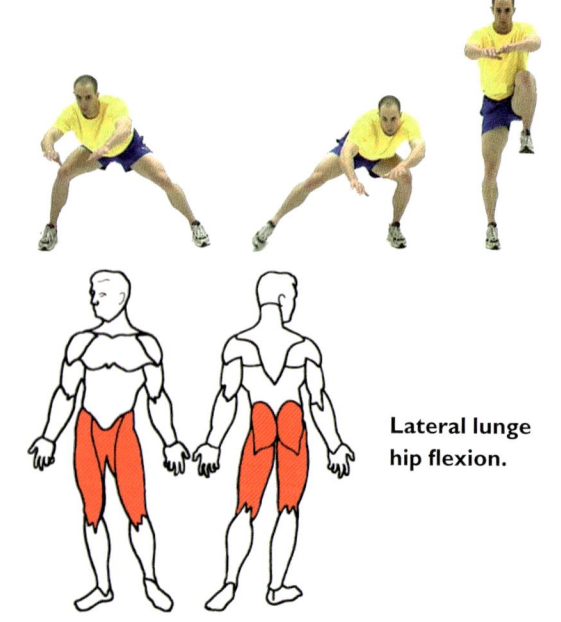

Lateral lunge hip flexion.

CASE STUDIES: THE PRACTICAL APPLICATION OF CORE CONDITIONING

- The movements are the same, as though stepping under and over an object. You can use hurdles/cones.
- The position of the step and the depth of the lunge can vary depending on the requirements of the exercise.
- The knees should track in line with the centre of the feet during the lunge.
- This exercise can be used as part of a warm-up, so gradually increase the speed and range of movements.

Caution: do not allow the knees to buckle in.

HIP EXTERNAL ROTATION STRETCH

2 × 6–8 left and right side.
Use a band or hands to assist the stretch.

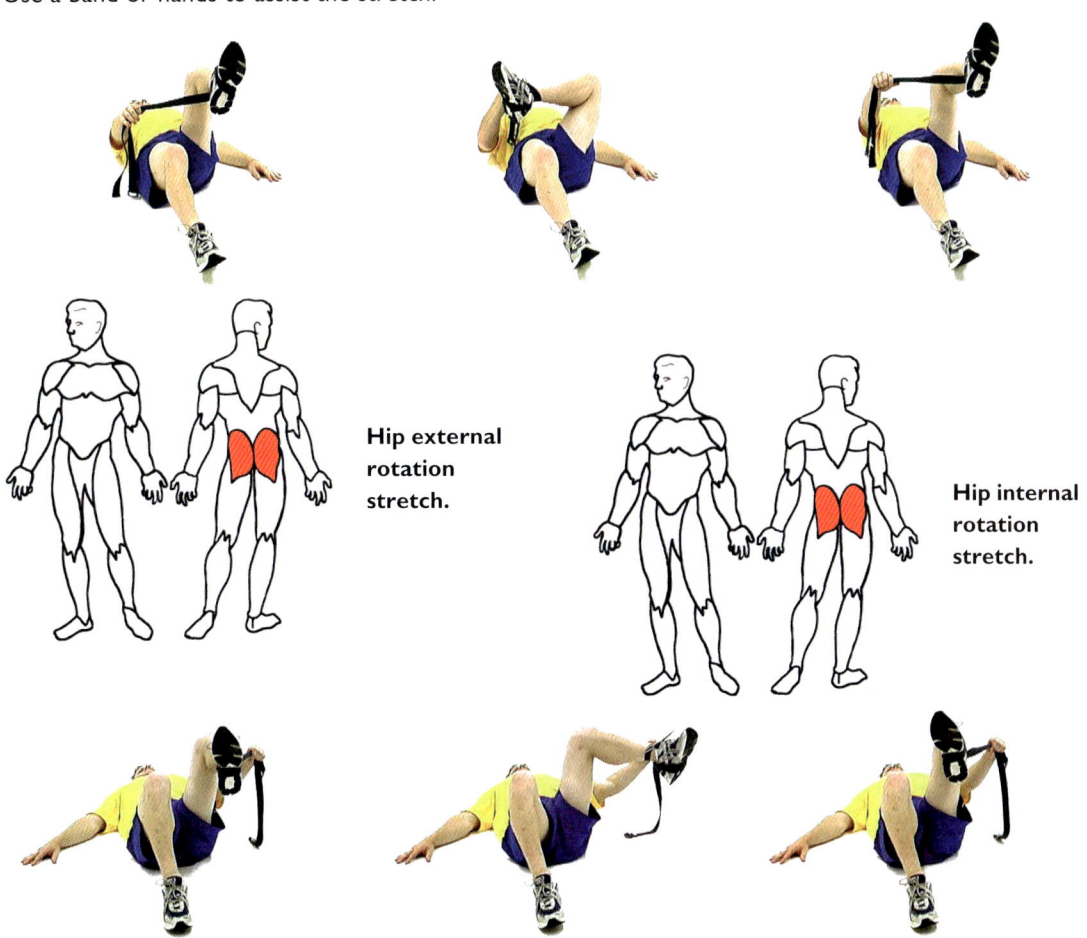

- Keep the thigh perpendicular to the ground and place the other hand on the knee to stabilize the leg if need be.
- Externally rotate the hip and pull further to increase the stretch as the external rotator muscles continue to contract.
- The duration of the stretch should be short, then repeat the process.

Caution: keep the head and shoulders relaxed and in contact with the ground.

HIP INTERNAL ROTATION STRETCH

2 × 6–8 left and right side.
Use a band or hands to assist the stretch.

Hip external rotation stretch.

Hip internal rotation stretch.

CASE STUDIES: THE PRACTICAL APPLICATION OF CORE CONDITIONING

- Keep the thigh perpendicular to the ground and place the other hand on the knee to stabilize the leg.
- Internally rotate the hip and pull further to increase the stretch as the internal rotator muscles continue to contract.
- The duration of the stretch should be short, then repeat the process.

Caution: keep the head and shoulders relaxed and in contact with the ground.

DOUBLE-LEG BRIDGING ON TO BENCH WITH ISOMETRIC BALL SQUEEZE BETWEEN KNEES

6 x 5-second holds x 3 total sets.
20 seconds rest in between sets.
Progress to feet on a Swiss ball to add some instability/further challenge.

- Position the feet securely on the bench with the hands on the floor.
- Lift the hips off the floor until the knees are at 90 degrees of flexion.
- Place a ball (football, rugby ball, light med ball) between your knees and squeeze tight as you hold.

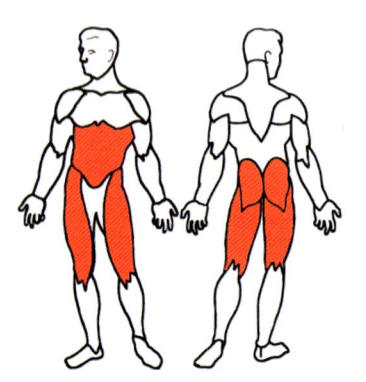

Double-leg bridging on to bench with isometric ball squeeze.

- Hold the position for 5 seconds.
- Lower to return to the start position, maintaining bent knees ready for the next repetition (5-second hold).
- Vary the position of the hands on the floor to assist with balance or place them across the chest to progress the difficulty of the exercise.

Caution: do not raise the body too high off the floor.

CONDITIONING SESSION

To be completed after the hip mobility warm-up/preparation. Select 6–7 out of 9 exercises to complete. Vary the selection in each session.

SINGLE-LEG BRIDGING

3 x 8 Left and right side.
Work alternate leg.

- Start with the feet approximately shoulder width apart, with the head and shoulders in contact with the ground.
- Lift the hips off the ground until the thighs are in line with the torso.
- Then lift one leg up and straight out, in line with your body.
- Hold for 2–3 seconds, and then control the movements back to the start position.

SPLIT SQUAT

3 sets x 12 repetitions left and right side.
Work alternate leg: minimal rest in between (feel the burn!).

- Assume a split stance with the hips and shoulders square and facing forward.

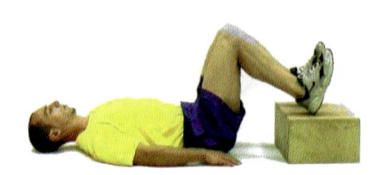

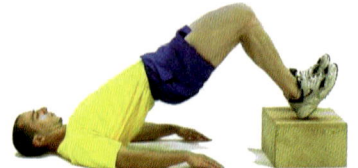

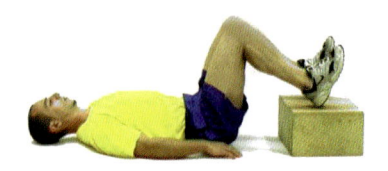

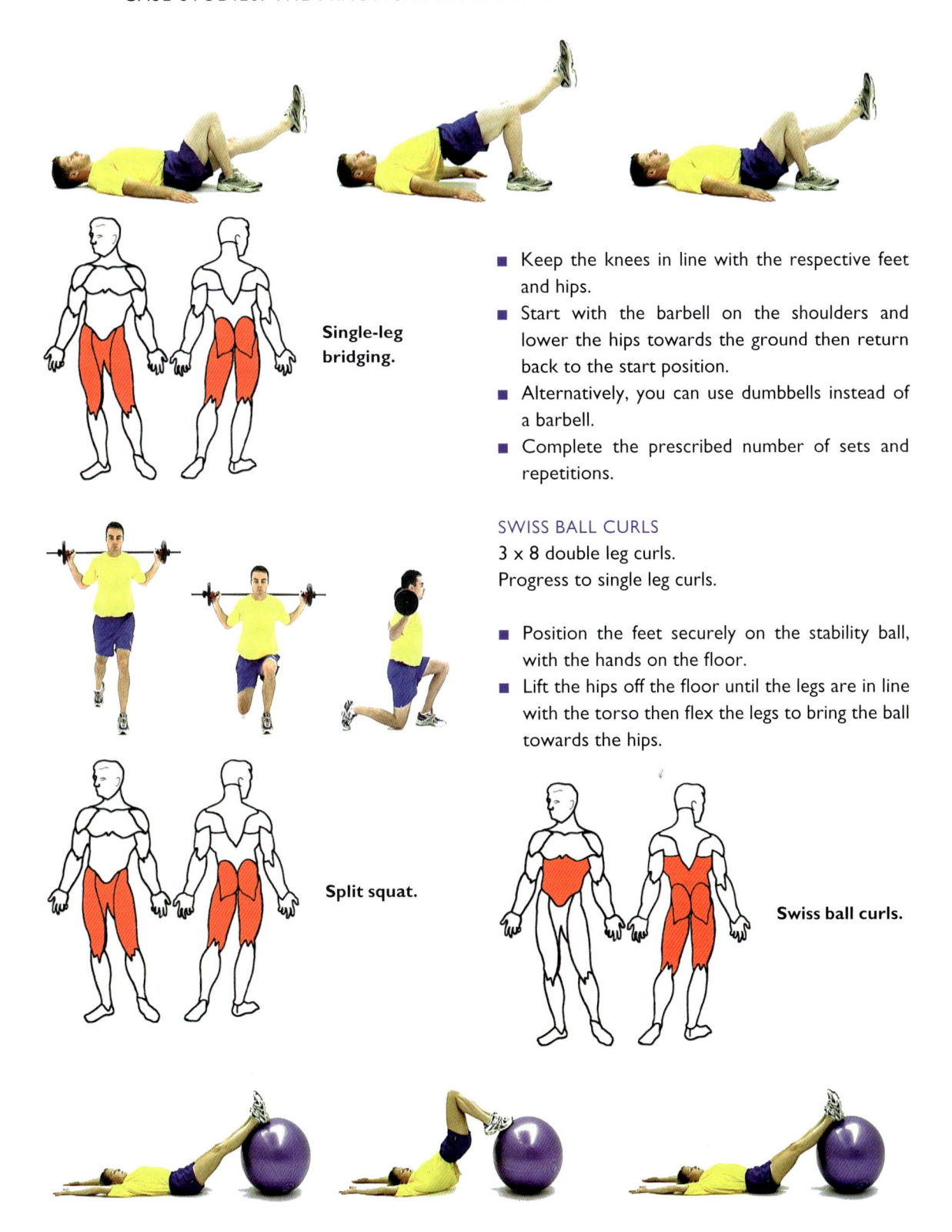

CASE STUDIES: THE PRACTICAL APPLICATION OF CORE CONDITIONING

Single-leg bridging.

- Keep the knees in line with the respective feet and hips.
- Start with the barbell on the shoulders and lower the hips towards the ground then return back to the start position.
- Alternatively, you can use dumbbells instead of a barbell.
- Complete the prescribed number of sets and repetitions.

SWISS BALL CURLS

3 x 8 double leg curls.
Progress to single leg curls.

- Position the feet securely on the stability ball, with the hands on the floor.
- Lift the hips off the floor until the legs are in line with the torso then flex the legs to bring the ball towards the hips.

Split squat.

Swiss ball curls.

CASE STUDIES: THE PRACTICAL APPLICATION OF CORE CONDITIONING

- Return back to the start position.
- Return to the floor after each repetition.
- As you get stronger, keep the body off the floor after each repetition.
- Vary the position of the hands on the floor to assist with balance, or place them across the chest to progress the difficulty of the exercise.

Caution: do not raise the body too high off the floor.

LATERAL STEP-UP WITH HIP FLEXION
3 x 12 left and right side.
Work alternate leg.

- The leg should be at 90 degrees when the foot is placed on the box.
- Complete with body weight to begin with.
- Side-step straight on to the box and raise/flex the following leg up with good mechanics as if you were running.
- With control, return to the start position.
- Complete the prescribed number of repetitions on one leg then switch sides.
- As you become more confident and stronger you can increase the distance from the box, to increase the challenge and adductor involvement.
- The height of the box should be so that your knee is at 90 degrees as you begin the exercise.

Caution: ensure that the box is stable and do not allow the knees to buckle in as you step up.

LATERAL LUNGE STEP-DOWN WITH WOOD-CHOP ROTATION
Can be completed on a BOSU as well.
3 x 8 left and right side.
Work alternate leg with quality and look after your back: brace and ensure good posture ('branding').

- Start with the medicine ball above the shoulder, with the torso in a slightly rotated position.
- Step sideways off the box and take the medicine ball across the body towards the outside of the leg, then push back firmly to the start position.

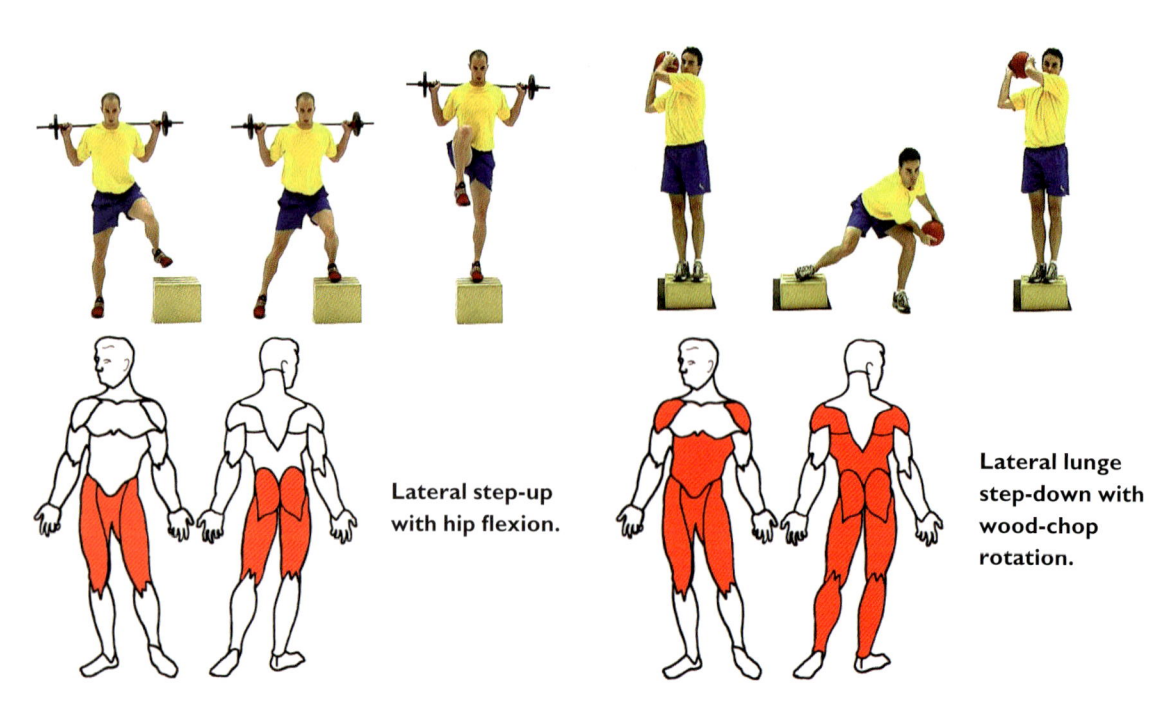

Lateral step-up with hip flexion.

Lateral lunge step-down with wood-chop rotation.

CASE STUDIES: THE PRACTICAL APPLICATION OF CORE CONDITIONING

- Land on the ground with a heel to toe stride. The flexion should be distributed through the leg, hip and the torso.
- The box height should be low to begin with (shin height).

Caution: ensure that the box is stable and not too high

MEDICINE BALL LUNGE ROTATION
3 x 8 left and right side.
Vary the lunge movement pattern to include straight lunges and diagonal lunge patterns.
30 seconds rest in between each set.

- Lunge and rotate the medicine ball across the body then push firmly to the start position.
- The knees should track in line with the centre of the feet during the lunge.
- Keep the hips and shoulders square and do not sway the torso forward or back.
- Rotate at your thoracic spine and use your obliques to complete the movement.

- A dumbbell or weights plate may be used as an alternative form of resistance.

Caution: do not allow the front knee to travel past the position of the foot. Perform with excellent control.

STRAIGHT-LEG ROMANIAN DEAD LIFT
4 x 8 repetitions.
Tempo: count of 3 to 4 down (eccentric phase) and 2 back up.
Strong back position/brace. Do no tilt through your spine.

- Assume a parallel stance with the hands wide on the barbell.
- Begin with the bar close to the shins with the arms straight and the shoulders over the bar.
- Keep the chest up and look forward or slightly up, with neutral curves in the spine.
- Flex at the hips until the bar travels below the knees, then extend the hips to reverse the movement back to the start position.

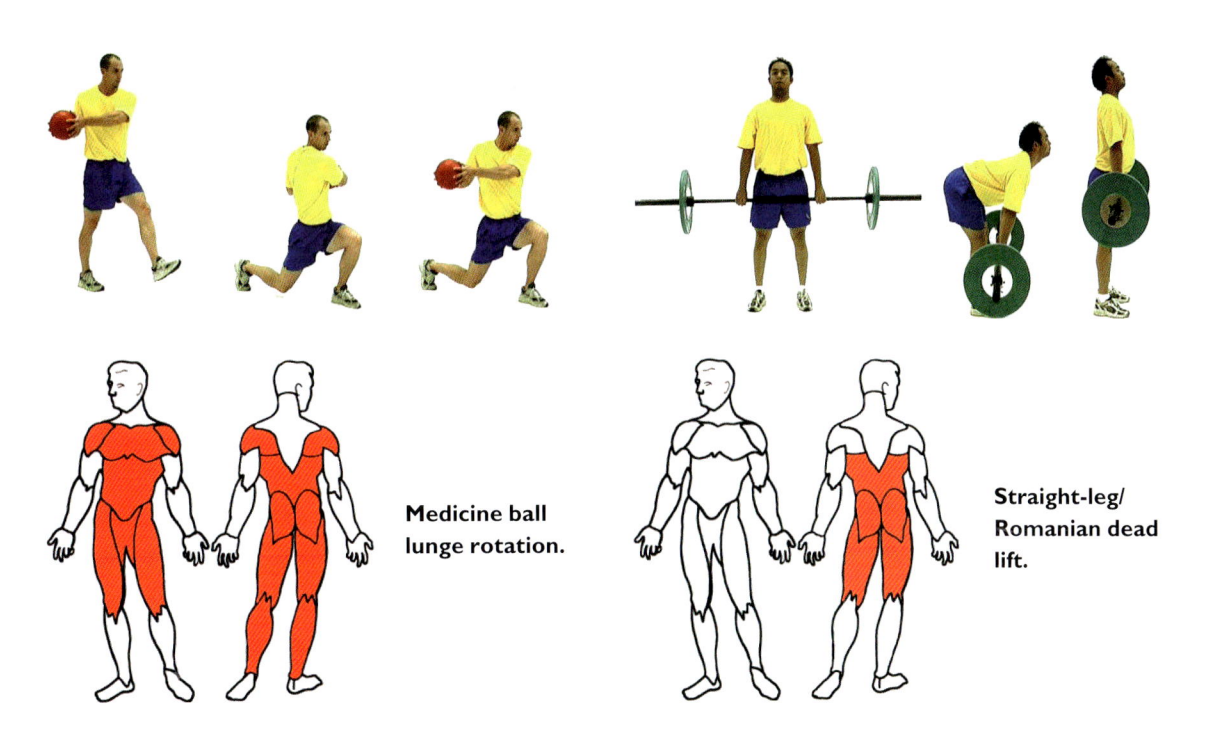

Medicine ball lunge rotation.

Straight-leg/Romanian dead lift.

105

CASE STUDIES: THE PRACTICAL APPLICATION OF CORE CONDITIONING

- Complete the prescribed number of sets and repetitions.

Caution: do not flex the spine or allow the shoulders to round. Do not allow the hips to rise before the shoulders.

CABLE HIP FLEXION, EXTENSION AND ABDUCTION/ADDUCTION CIRCUIT

Complete a circuit with variations as follows:

- Hip flexion and extension (kicking movement).
- Abduction and adduction (side pass movement).

3 x 12 of each movement as a circuit.
Rest on alternate leg (work both sides).

- Place a cable or a band around the ankle/lower limb.
- Take a step away to allow for some resistance on the cable/band.
- Control both phases of the movement.
- Complete one of the prescribed movement patterns: side-step turn and flex/kick; extend and flex; full range-of-movement hip extension and kick movement.
- Vary the movement patterns to include all ranges of movement with the cable or band,

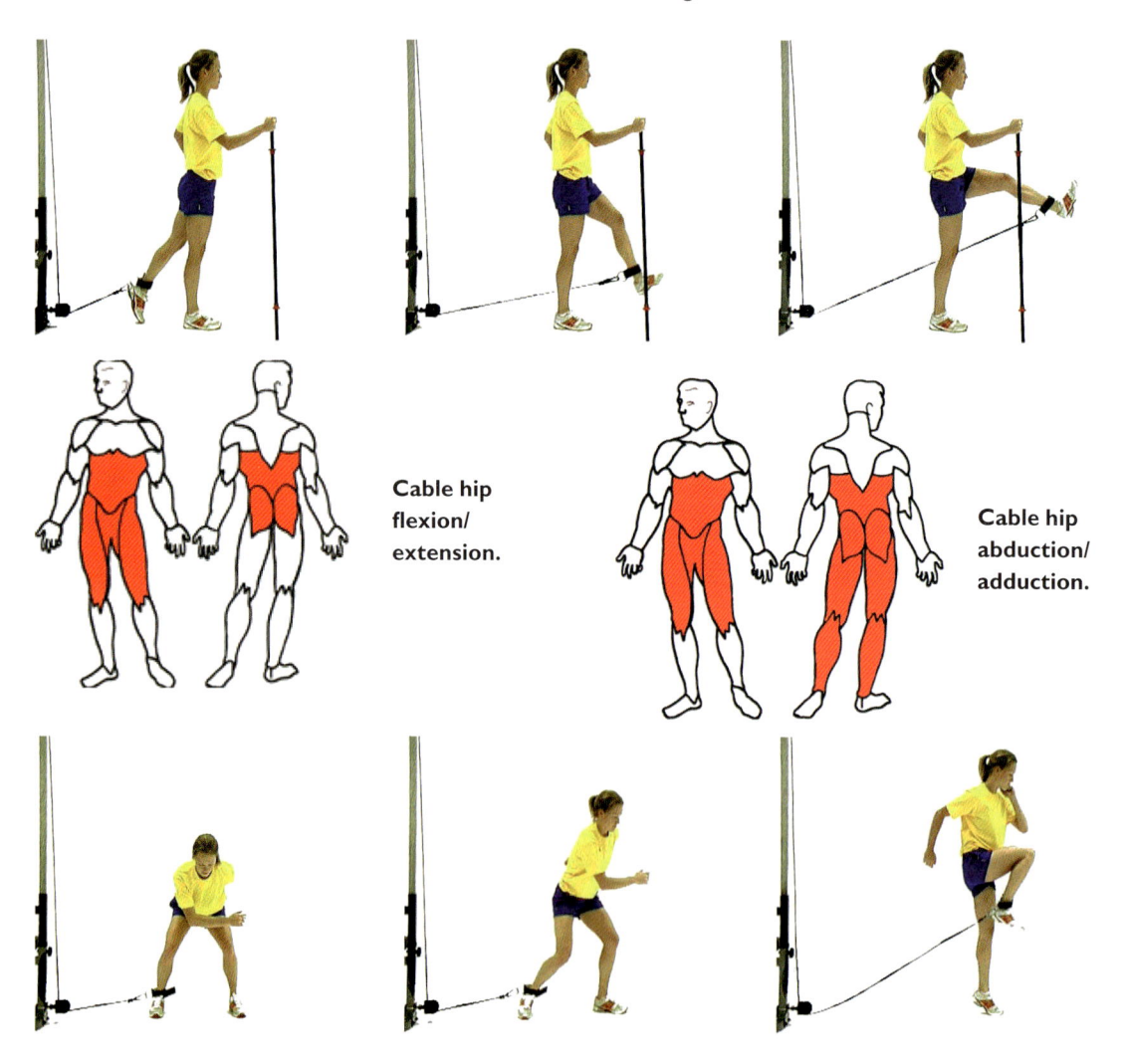

Cable hip flexion/extension.

Cable hip abduction/adduction.

CASE STUDIES: THE PRACTICAL APPLICATION OF CORE CONDITIONING

always maintaining a good position and bracing through the core.

Caution: ensure that the cable or band is firmly attached. Stay braced through the core to ensure a strong movement pattern and encourage good mechanics.

MULTI-DIRECTIONAL LUNGES

(Clock lunges: 12 o'clock, 2 o'clock, 3 o'clock and 5 o'clock)
3 rotations at 4 clock positions: 12 o'clock, 2 o'clock, 3 o'clock and 5 o'clock, left and right leg (lots of volume).
Rest = 30 seconds.
Repeat x 3 total sets.
Progress overhead load (as per the image).

- Lunge forward to 12 o'clock.
- Then push firmly off the front leg back to the start position.
- Then lunge to 2 o'clock and push back to the start position.
- Repeat to 3 o'clock and 5 o'clock.
- Switch legs.
- Flex at the hips and maintain good posture ('branding') during the descent of each of the lunges.
- The knee should track in line with the centre of the foot.
- Do not allow the knee to buckle in or twist.

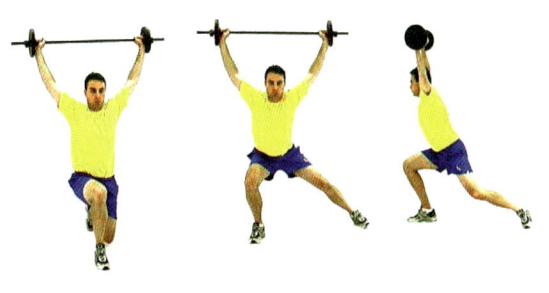

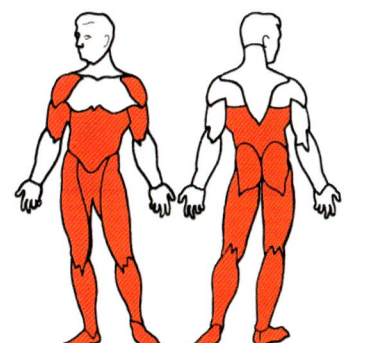

Additional/Supplementary Conditioning Exercises

Introduced and varied/progressed over the 8 weeks during which I saw the client (see overleaf).

Progressions

Exercises were progressed as follows:

- The client had a reasonable level of baseline conditioning from being generally active.
- He had never been injured so reassuring him that he would become a better athlete as a result of some specific rehab was important.
- Familiarity with the hip mobility exercises took about 2 weeks. He had his favourite exercises but I encouraged him to complete a combination of the options. This became habitual before he did any other exercise and took about 10 minutes once he was familiar with it.
- The strength programme worked well for him and he really bought into the plan.
- Most exercises were very functional: addressing his injury, general strength and core/posterior chain.
- Load was increased regularly, and the client worked to a repetition maximum for most strength exercises.
- Exercise RPE progressed from 2–3 (easy–moderate) and as his confidence and function improved he worked up to 8–9 (very, very hard).

Multi-directional lunges.

CASE STUDIES: THE PRACTICAL APPLICATION OF CORE CONDITIONING

Exercise	Sets x reps and rest	Rationale	Comments
Dead lift	4 x 8 reps 45 seconds rest in between	Strength and power development. Functional movement.	Progressed well and enjoyed the feel of a loaded bar. Technique was good.
Proprioception	4 x 20 seconds L and R leg Work alternate leg	Always an important addition to any rehab plan: encouraged good posture, kicking ball, passing ball etc. during proprioception exercises.	Likes the involvement of a ball. Used a football and kicking as rehab progressed, which he enjoyed.
High pull (from a hang position)	4 x 8 repetitions 45 seconds rest	Functional exercise, very good for endurance capacity and local muscular fatigue. Whole body exercise.	Needed to coach the movement pattern but once familiar the client liked this exercise. Progress load well.
Speed, agility and quickness (SAQ)	8- to 12-minute session on local football pitch. Duration of session and intensity progressed as rehab progressed.	Football-specific movement patterns introduced once a good foundation of straight-line movement achieved. Progress to lateral movements with control then more dynamic and reactive. Then increase in intensity, acceleration, deceleration and introducing a ball.	Progressed the intensity over the weeks to high intensity (RPE = 7–8) to include multi-directional/football-specific movement patterns in and out of ladders, zig-zags, acceleration, deceleration work. Performed and progressed well with confidence and function. Included a ball out of the exercises: passing drills and dribbling, etc.
Kettle bell swings	3 x 12 repetitions 30 seconds rest in between sets.	Dynamic movement, which encourages explosively extending the body but with good core and glute/pelvic control at full extension. Encouraged quite a wide stance to activate adductors. Required a combination of good control and explosive movement for the exercise.	A good addition to the programme. Progressed it from completing only the repetitions to super setting it with some lateral movements and acceleration work after each set.
Football-specific conditioning work	Built up the duration from 5 minutes introductory to 20–30 minutes higher-intensity ball work.	Functional conditioning and fitness work to prepare for a return to play.	Progressed from one-touch small passes, to two-touch to higher-intensity box drills and passing and crossing the ball. Two of the client's team mates joined us towards the end of his rehabilitation programme to help progress the passing and functional work.

CASE STUDIES: THE PRACTICAL APPLICATION OF CORE CONDITIONING

Progressions of exercise selection:

- Foundation exercises were completed initially, and the complexity and challenge progressed over time.
- Lateral movement patterns were introduced with good control from week one with me, as the client had been completing isometric early rehab work with the physiotherapist before being passed on to work with me. This meant that he had a good isometric strength base and I could then progress with concentric and eccentric work at a higher level.
- More dynamic functional work was introduced over the weeks and a return-to-running plan was provided by me. This was an 8-week functional plan to complement the strength programme, with the aim of allowing the client to return to play after a thorough rehabilitation.
- Early on, the client also complemented his strength and hip mobility work with pool work and bike/off-feet conditioning work and upper body strength.
- The pool work included running in the pool and multi-directional movement patterns, including some of the standing hip mobility work: open the gate, close the gate and internal/external rotation.
- The client had pool access via his gym membership, which became very useful.

Outcome

- I saw the client initially 3 weeks in a row then every 2–3 weeks thereafter.
- The client wasn't particularly happy to be injured but after discussion he recognized the importance of a thorough rehabilitation programme and I assured him that he would be a better, more robust athlete as a result of the rehabilitation.
- The client was able to increase the session intensity RPE over the weeks, progressing from an initial prescription of 2–3 (easy–moderate) to 4–5 (moderate to hard). By the end of the programme, he managed to work to a capacity of around 8–9 (very, very hard).
- The client's capacity to work at a high intensity increased. His overall fitness was improved, and he was much stronger as a result of the plan.
- The global movement patterns and strength work, which included the sling systems, posterior chain and core, helped the client become more robust.
- The physiotherapist was delighted with his presentation after the programme and was very happy to return him to play.
- Strength and conditioning has become part of the client's regular week now and he is enjoying his football more than ever before.

CASE STUDY SUMMARY

These six different case studies tell the story of clients who have all benefited from improved lumbo-pelvic hip strength, core strength and general lower limb strength and, consequently, have improved their function. All cases progressed from isometric conditioning to more dynamic movement patterning with load, to varying degrees and demands. The link from the sling system, core and posterior chain in many of these movement patterns highlights the requirement for global conditioning, to complement isolated strengthening at the early stages. This dovetails with general conditioning to help prepare the client for a return to play or pain-free activity.

It would be remiss of an S&C coach to fail to address the global muscles within a programme, and to focus only on the core musculature. The rehabilitation or reconditioning of the client is a journey back to function, and this should be considered within the exercise prescription. Considering isolation exercises only, when the body moves as a whole unit, would be wrong in the long run. Sometimes, of course, isolated exercises may be prescribed – in the early stages of rehabilitation, this is often the case – but it is essential for an S&C practitioner to put in place a whole-body programme. This is done by looking at how the body moves, completing the needs analysis for the individual, considering their training history, injury history, time commitments, facility availability and goals, and to provide a programme that ensures that the body moves well and with function, and that those goals are met. For example, in order to progress to pain-free movement whilst walking, it makes sense to strengthen the lower limbs in addition to strengthening the core and lower back, if there is a history of prolapsed disc.

Within these case studies there is a high volume of different exercises for each client – often 8–10 in each client's programme – in order to introduce a varying amount of stimulus, which will help with adaptation, muscle memory and exposure to loading patterns. As things improve, the programme can be fine-tuned and adjusted. The needs analysis may be reassessed once the initial problem has been addressed and maybe 4–5 specific exercises can be fine-tuned to continue the progress of the individual. However, if the desired stimulus can be achieved in 4–5 exercises from the start, then I will prescribe 4–5 exercises! Everything is prescribed for an outcome and with purpose and is flexible, of course.

A few weeks or months into the programme, if the client has adhered well to the plan and has not experienced any setbacks, his or her focus will move from rehabilitation to normal daily activity again, such as returning to running a 10k or playing football, or enjoying day-to-day activities pain-free. The conditioning programme is fluid and, rather like a pendulum, may swing to and from certain areas at the appropriate time. The programme can change over time as an individual progresses and adapts. The above case studies offer an insight into the first initial strength and conditioning intervention in the early weeks after specialist referral or self-referral. Thereafter, once some training adaptation has begun (normally after 6–8 weeks), the programme will evolve. This is done by manipulation of the sets, repetitions, intensity and load, in addition to exercise selection. It is important to stick with the programme to allow adaptation but also to manipulate the body's stimulus regularly, as in every strength programme.

I always explain to my athletes or clients that, despite their injury, I am convinced that, if they follow their plan, they will come out the other side stronger and more robust, with better body awareness. It should allow them to enjoy a lifetime of sport and activity. As people live longer, surely a focus on strength and wellbeing while an individual is young and more capable, creating a good foundation of strength, will improve their quality of life in their later years. It is a worthwhile investment of time. Not everything can be prevented, but certainly by addressing any weaknesses and becoming stronger, the body's resilience will be improved. The successful outcomes from these case studies are surely evidence that being stronger can make life better and protect the body over the years.

CHAPTER 4

APPLIED CORE CONDITIONING: PROGRAMMING, PRESCRIPTION AND SPORTS-SPECIFIC TRAINING

The exercises prescribed in the case studies should provide a number of solutions to some real-life issues. They illustrate how it is possible functionally to apply the principles of strength and conditioning to strengthening the core and associated musculature. The philosophy that the body works as a whole unit is really important in this functional exercise concept. It is important that the practitioner applying the principles recognizes that the core may be trained and conditioned in a multitude of ways – prone laying, supine, standing, kneeling, single-leg, double-leg, and so on – and by using a variety of equipment, such as Swiss balls, BOSU, cables, medicine balls, mini bands, dumbbells, barbells and benches. It all adds to the challenge and stimulus.

The key to success is using the needs analysis to consider the whole picture. Planning a programme or intervention is individual to each client, and yet there will be a crossover from the various exercises that may work from one client to the next. The trick is to make these choices relevant and applicable to each particular client's requirements.

Most people I see, even high-level sports people who are generally well conditioned, can all benefit, for example, from single-leg bridging, as the posterior chain is often neglected. That exercise, like many others, also allows for a number of progressions, from basic single-leg bridging to using a Swiss ball, varying the position of the arms, changing the speed of movement and tempo, or the numbers of sets and repetitions, loading bi-laterally or unilaterally, with a weight plate or dumbbell, to increasing instability by using a BOSU, balance cushion or foam roller to lie on, kneel on or step on to – and so on, and so on. An exercise can be progressed in many, many ways, or it may be necessary to move on to something more challenging, to ensure the body has increased stimulus. In the case of single-leg bridging, for example, the client may progress to loaded hip thrusts once a good foundation has been achieved. Many athletes focus on their anterior conditioning, their 'beach' muscles, and forget to address their posterior chain strength. Of course, many of the injuries seen at the highest level can be caused by a number of factors. However, ensuring that the core strength, lumbo-pelvic hip strength and sling systems are immense will surely be protective.

APPLIED CORE CONDITIONING: PROGRAMMING, PRESCRIPTION

The way in which the programme is planned and prescribed can significantly affect the outcome. Below are some guidelines in programming and prescription, followed by some sport-specific exercises to address the areas around the core and make the individual stronger relative to the demands placed upon them by their sport.

PROGRAMMING AND PRESCRIPTION

Progressive loading during rehabilitation and general conditioning is important, as well as smart exercise selection. A foundation needs to be created then progressed. Depending on what level the client or athlete is at when they see you, their injury history, any pain and what their goals and time scales are will depend on what you prescribe. The foundation and progression should move from isometric exercises to exercises involving concentric and eccentric loading.

Isometric Strength

In isometric exercises, the muscle is activated, but, instead of being allowed to lengthen or shorten, it is held at a constant length and contracted. These exercises are used for early-stage rehabilitation and foundation core strength and development. They are also good for improving body awareness in individuals who are unfamiliar with conditioning and loading the body. They are especially useful during acute injury and rehabilitation.

With isometric exercises the core can remain still and contracted but, for example, a limb can move. In addition, the core or posterior chain can just be held in a contracted isometric position without any limb moving. This is why this can be an effective way to condition the core when injured or in pain. The individual can learn to brace and activate the muscles, use their breathing and activate. Because there is no movement there should be no pain. These exercises should always be used in an early-stage rehabilitation setting. They provide an excellent way for the individual to gain confidence as they progress and become stronger. They can then progress to more challenging dynamic movements as strength and control improve.

Examples of specific foundation isometric core exercises are shown below:

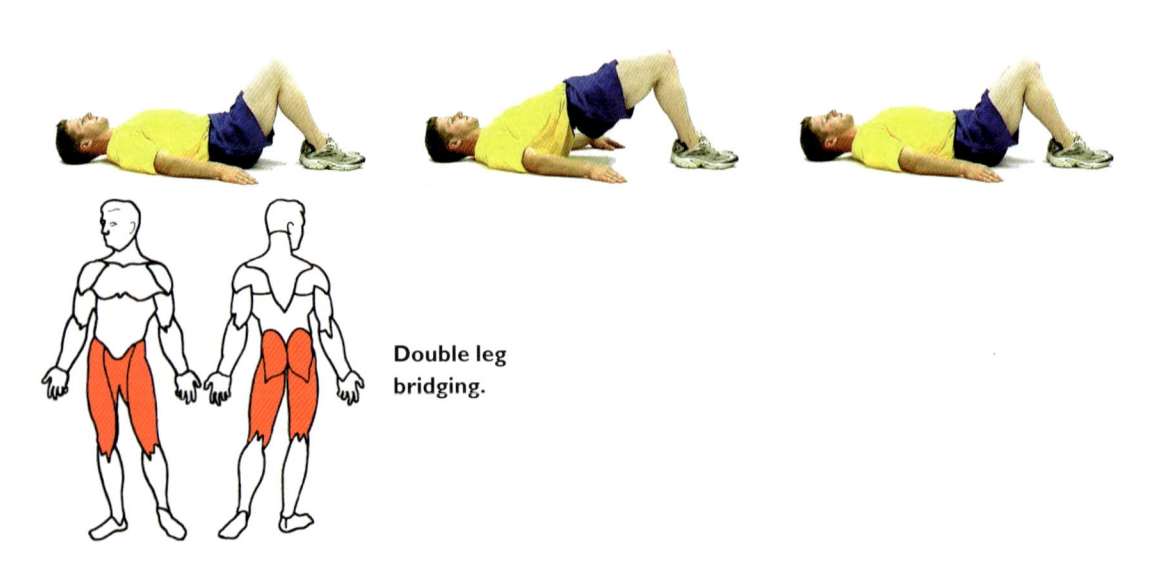

Double leg bridging.

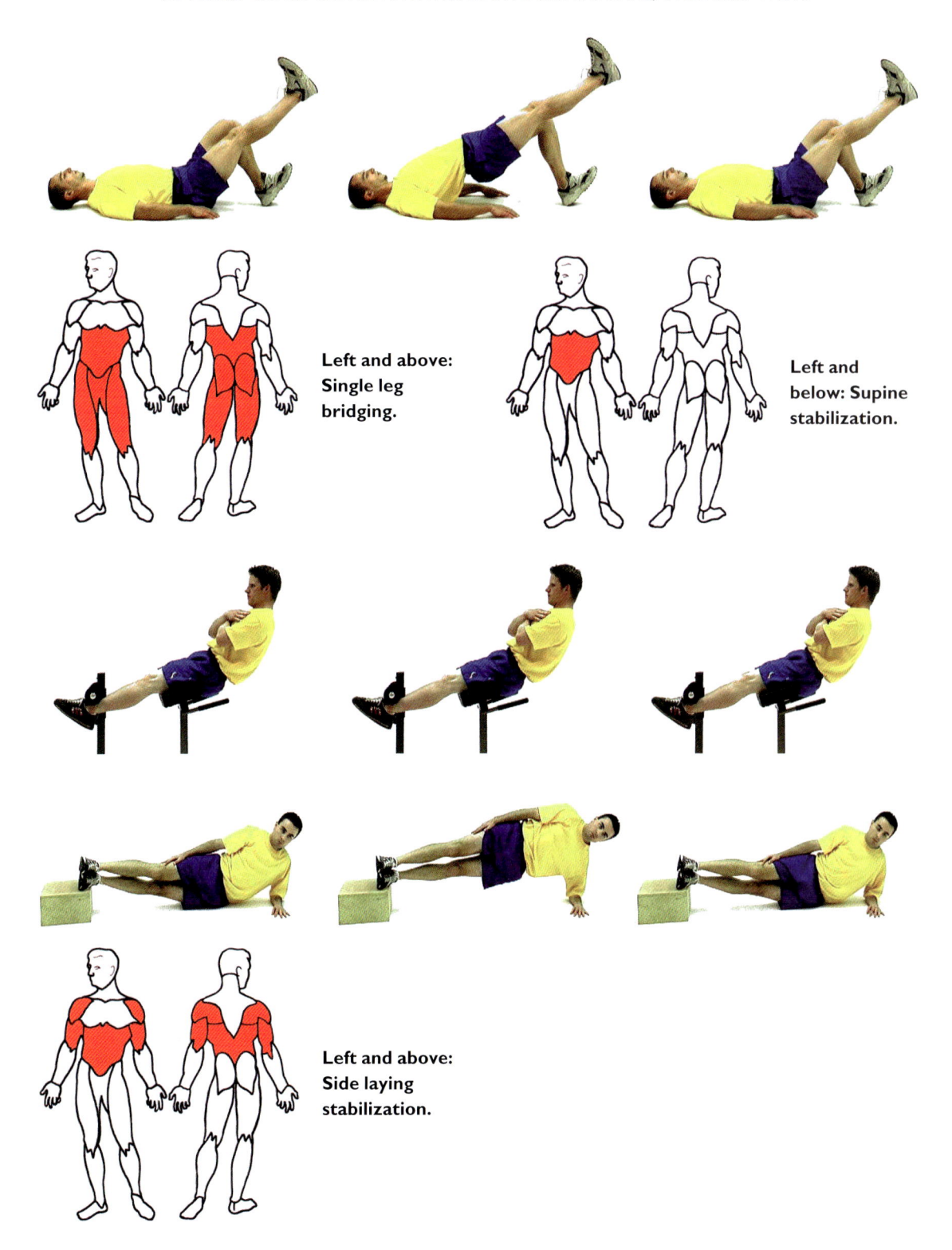

APPLIED CORE CONDITIONING: PROGRAMMING, PRESCRIPTION

Left and above: Single leg bridging.

Left and below: Supine stabilization.

Left and above: Side laying stabilization.

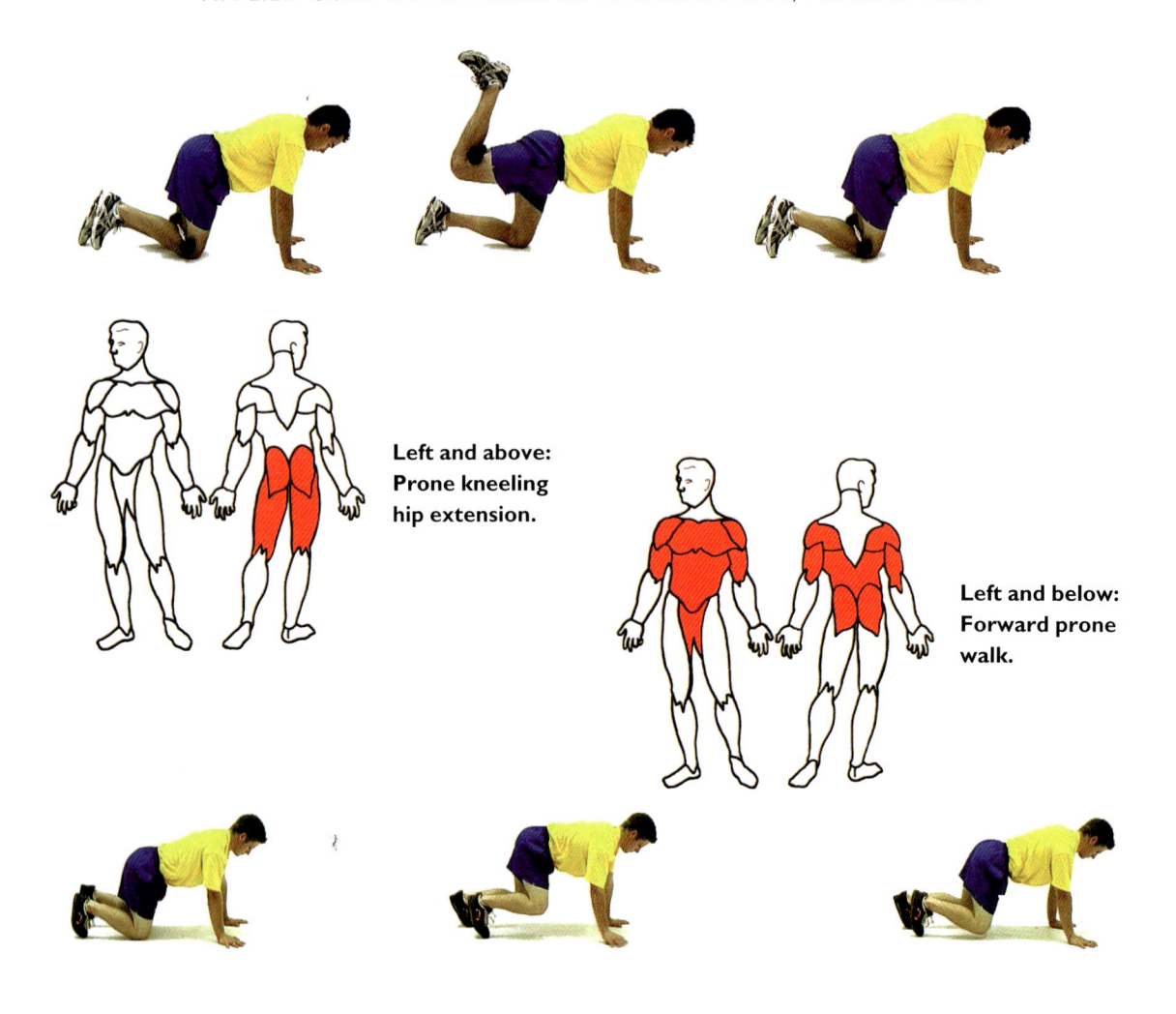

APPLIED CORE CONDITIONING: PROGRAMMING, PRESCRIPTION

Left and above: Prone kneeling hip extension.

Left and below: Forward prone walk.

Concentric and Eccentric Loading: Dynamic Progressions with Control

As things progress and the individual becomes stronger, new challenges can be presented. This is where additional load, angles and movement in different planes around the body can be introduced. The individual will have mastered the bracing and breathing by now, so that it occurs almost instinctively and subconsciously. At this stage, external forces can be applied, using cables, mini bands, medicine balls, Swiss balls, weight plates, and so on. To be honest, the only limitation is the imagination.

The main rule is that everything still has to be performed with control – movements can be chaotic but it must be a controlled chaos! When the quality of movement suffers due to fatigue, the individual should rest and recover, and then go again once they have recovered. A determination to complete an activity to extend the body's capacity is important for progress, but it must always be done with an attention to detail. Form can be held as long as possible for overload to occur, but not at the cost of poor technique. These movements can be eccentric or concentric in nature.

Examples of dynamic progressions are shown below:

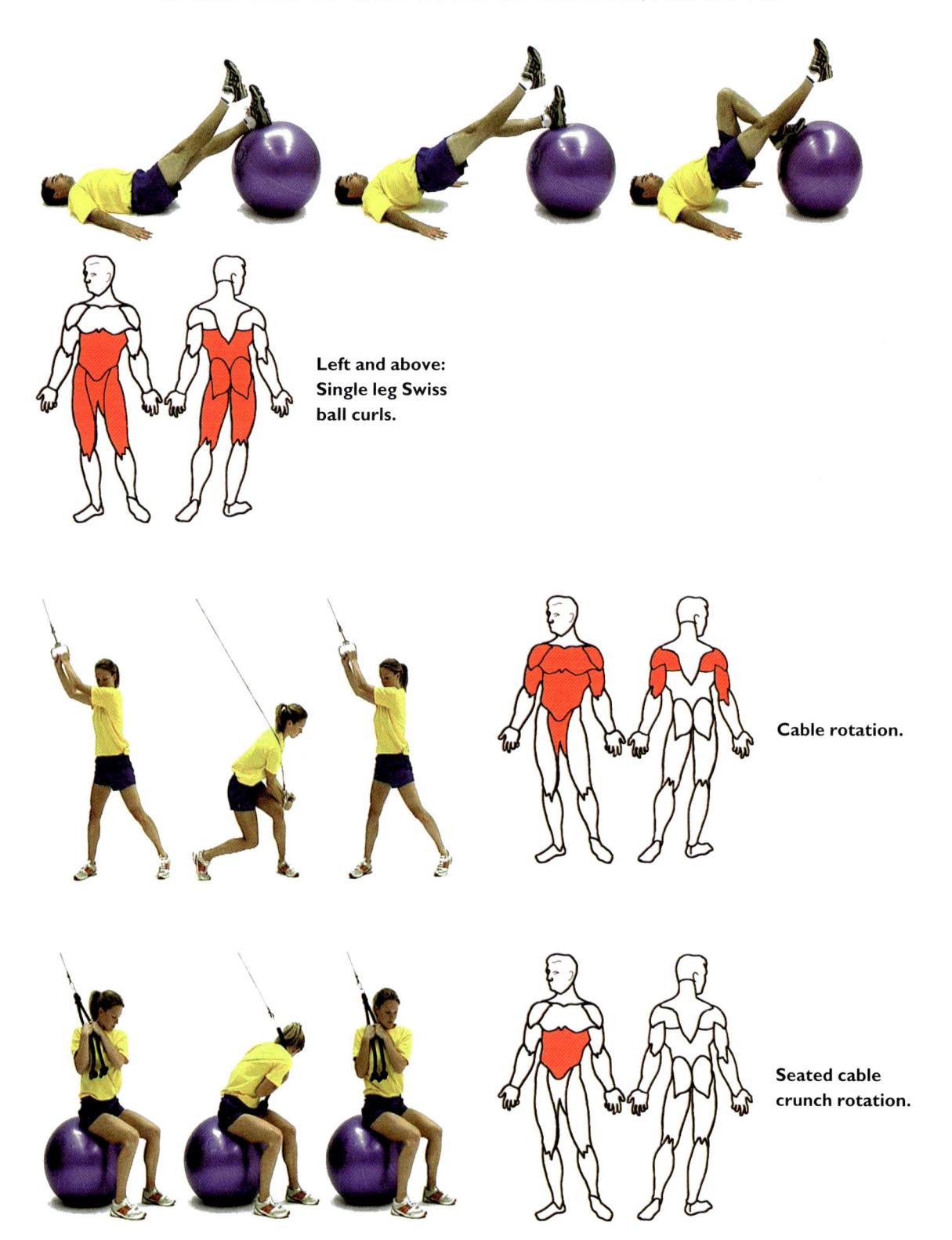

APPLIED CORE CONDITIONING: PROGRAMMING, PRESCRIPTION

Left and above: Single leg Swiss ball curls.

Cable rotation.

Seated cable crunch rotation.

115

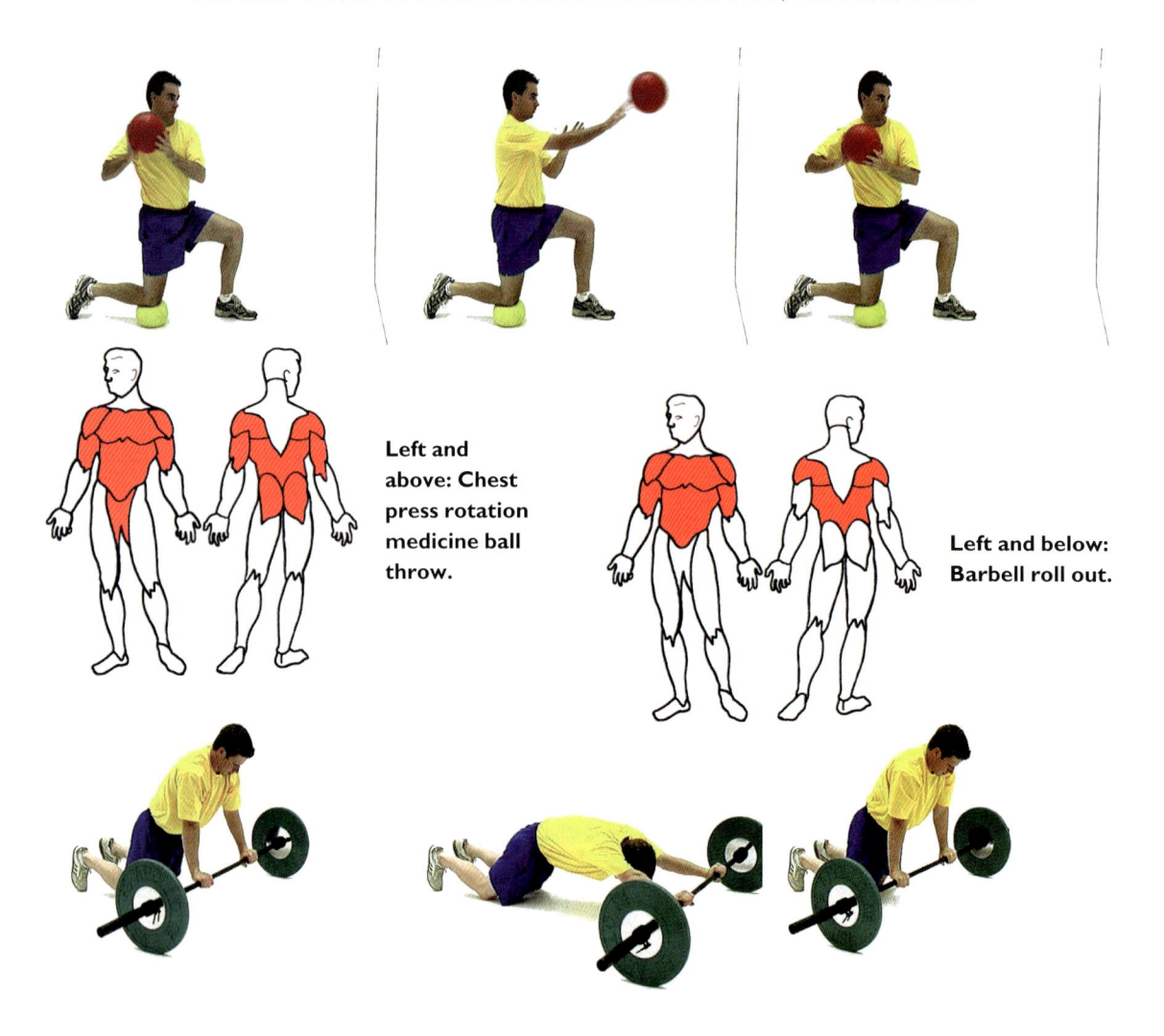

Left and above: Chest press rotation medicine ball throw.

Left and below: Barbell roll out.

SPORT SPECIFIC-TRAINING AND PRESCRIPTION OPTIONS

A comprehensive applied core conditioning programme is an excellent addition to an overall training programme that incorporates multi-joint exercises, Olympic lifts and free weights, as demonstrated in the case studies and supplemental assistance exercises described earlier.

Gottschall et al. (2013) completed research with the purpose of evaluating the muscle activity of distal and proximal muscles during a series of both isolation and integration exercises. They hypothesized that isolation exercises would elicit greater activity of the primary abdominal and lumbar muscles compared with integrated exercises. The results, however, demonstrated the opposite – that the activation of the abdominal and lumbar muscles was greatest during the integration exercises that required activation of deltoid and gluteal muscles. This demonstrated the importance of more whole-body activities, to optimize core activation. It is important for an S&C practitioner to remember this when prescribing exercises aimed at strengthening the core, and achieving rehabilitation and improved performance.

Arokoski *et al.* (2001) also compared abdominal and erector spinae activity during exercises with and without a balance component. In one example, the participants completed a bridge exercise with both feet on the ground and then with one leg lifted. The average electromyographic amplitude was at least 20 per cent greater in the rectus abdominus, longissimus thoracis and multifidus muscles with one leg lifted, and 200 per cent greater in the external oblique muscles than when both legs were on the floor. This shows how decreasing the stability of the exercise places higher demands on the core muscles, thereby increasing activation and improving the strength and stability of those muscles.

These progressions are important during exercise prescription and programme design. There should always be a purpose and a progression to each exercise, whether through loading, increasing sets and/or reps, or making the exercise less stable. However, increased instability sometimes leads to a compromise in terms of strength or power output, so a decision needs to be made by the practitioner regarding outcome goals for a particular exercise. An example would be to use double-leg bridging and progress to single-leg bridging, then bridging on a Swiss ball to increase the instability and activation demands. However, as the baseline strength improves for the athlete or client, it may be appropriate to transition into a more strength- and power-based activity and progress to a loaded hip thrust, using a barbell and developing more posterior strength and power. It would be remiss to do this before the foundation control and strength base had been achieved, but progressing to it over time is an appropriate prescription and design.

Research suggests that multi-joint exercises such as the squat, Romanian dead lift and good morning exercise stimulate greater muscle activation in the posterior chain core group than stability ball exercises training those same muscles (Nuzzo *et al.*, 2008). In addition, multi-joint free-weight exercises provide adequate stimulus to the lumbar multifidus, transverse abdominis and quadratus lumborum. This is good news for sports-specific conditioning and athletic development, which also require multi-joint exercises in coordination with excellent core strength.

Prescribing relative to the requirements and demands of the individual and their chosen sport is vital for success, along with the inclusion of graduated physiological overload. The key to a good programme is to keep things simple. First, the client needs to understand what is being asked of them, via verbal cues or visual demonstration. If they do not understand the exercise or the key target outcomes, they will not be able to perform it well. Under direction, they need to focus on excellent movement patterns, to ensure that there is no compromise on technique, especially when fatigued. They also need to ensure that they are being subjected to the right level of challenge and physiological overload, once pain has subsided and technique is good. Over time, the aim should be to progress effectively from single-plane movements that are isometric, to multi-plane movements, which become more dynamic movements with different muscular and neurological demands. Once a foundation of strength has been achieved, then the exercises can become more sports-specific, mimicking the type of movement that occurs during sport, varying the stance or position and increasing the load.

Volume and loading need to be well thought out, based upon the training experience of the individual as well as their current presentation: are they peaking for competition, so at a high level of conditioning, or are they recovering from injury? Or are they relatively new to training, with limited experience? The prescription and programme will depend very much on the answers to these questions.

Often, initially, body weight is enough stimulus for many exercises, for example, a plank hold or bridging. The key to successful prescription then is the sets, repetitions, rest and tempo of the movement. All four considerations will influence the eventual outcome. Sometimes, the tempo needs to be slow and controlled, to encourage activation and an isometric contraction for, say, a count of 3 or 4 seconds. Sometimes, it may be more dynamic, with a count of 1 or 2. This timing will change the feeling and sensation of the specific exercise and also the outcome: more endurance-based = higher tempo, more activation and control and also with eccentric demands the prescription would be with a slower tempo on the lowering phase.

Duration can also be specified, for example, a plank hold could be prescribed initially for 30 seconds, and the duration progressed over a few weeks as the individual adapts and becomes stronger. Once a level of strength has been achieved and the individual is competent, progressions can be introduced. In the case of the plank hold, an arm raise or leg raise, or some rotation, may be added within the 30-second hold, or the duration may be increased.

Isometric/Endurance-Based Exercise Example: Plank Hold

Sport-specific relevance: this an important foundation exercise that will be of value for every sport. It also plays a part in injury prevention or after acute injury, as the isometric contraction and lack of movement ensure that any pain is minimal. The plank hold is a prerequisite for future core training and development, lifting weights and intense exercise. It strengthens the core, glutes, low back and also the shoulders. Progressions are simple: increase duration, raise an arm, lift a leg, or complete on a BOSU, foam roller, balance cushion or Swiss ball. It really is a great foundation exercise that is easy to start and to assess, in terms of duration and improvement. It is also relevant to all activities, whether occupational, lifting at work or sports-specific.

Specific sports that can benefit: every sport will benefit from an inclusion of isometric plank holds and their progressions. It can be included as part of a foundation training programme for youths, sedentary population and athletes, as well as drivers, construction workers and health-care workers, for example.

There is no rush to achieve the high-level progressions given as examples here. Depending on the training experience (also known as training age), injury history and goals of the individual, certain markers will indicate to the strength and conditioning coach that it is time to progress. Sometimes, the same exercise may be amended to add stimulus, as in the suggestions here, while on other occasions a different exercise may be selected as a progression or for a different stimulus. It is not a race to get to the next level: it is about quality and control. I intentionally do not give too much rest during the endurance core sessions. The rationale is that the core musculature is being trained to cope with regular endurance-based demands. The essential point is that quality is always maintained. I would rather an individual stop and rest if their quality was

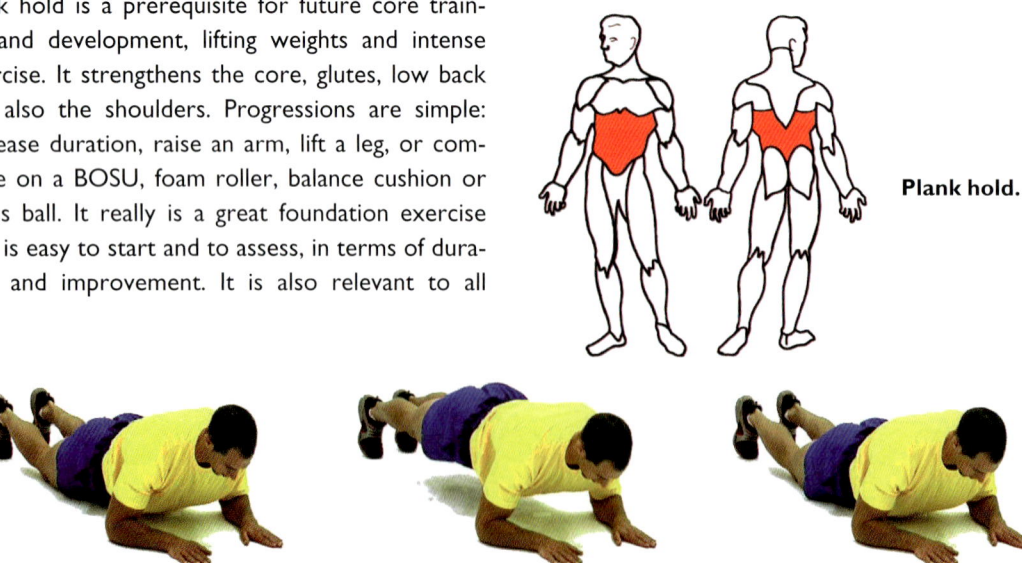

Plank hold.

Plank Hold

Plank hold	Sets and rest	Reps	Tempo	Frequency	Load	Progression
Level 1: Introductory	3–4 sets 10–20 seconds rest	20–30 second hold	Controlled/isometric-based	3–4 x each week	Body weight	Increased duration and quality of hold
Level 2: Body awareness developed – good strength progressions	3–4 sets 10–20 seconds rest	Consider increasing duration from 20–30 seconds onwards – increase by 5–10 seconds duration per session. Introduce alternate leg or arm lifts within duration of hold.	Controlled/isometric-based 30-second hold increasing duration as necessary to leg lift or arm lift: Tempo during limb lift = 2-3-2 with control.	3–4 x each week	Body weight and progression to external load by moving a limb (gravity) if capable whist maintaining excellent technique and position.	Increased duration and decreased contact with the ground. Increased load: moving a limb (gravity)
Level 3: Body awareness is excellent, and strength and control are developing well	3–4 sets 10–15 seconds rest Always quality work	30 seconds to >60 second holds Increased duration and progress loading with rotation movement, knee lifts as well as alternate leg/arm movements with load.	Progress to dynamic movement patterns and multi-planar movements. Tempo can vary to be quicker or slower to add to the challenge, but always maintaining excellent position and control.	3–4 x each week	External load: dumbbells, medicine ball, bands in addition to increased instability via BOSU, Swiss ball, suspension training, balance cushion, foam roller, etc.	Progress dynamic nature of exercise: add rotation, leg lift, arm lift, holding dumbbells, using a BOSU, Swiss ball, medicine ball, suspension training, foam roller or balance cushion to lean on or mini bands around hands to complete different movement patterns. Also crawler patterns are excellent for progression.
Level 4 and on-going	Consider on-going progressions but ensure quality movement patterns throughout. It is likely that the level achieved by dedicated work at this point will continue to be stimulated by the activities and external load progressions prescribed at level 3. Variations can be introduced.					

compromised with 10 seconds to go, rather than carry on for those last 10 seconds, but with poor control.

Coaching point: if needed, rest, recover and go again with quality.

Some practitioners would advise >60 seconds rest in between a plank hold, for example. In my view, this is too long – I want to create an overload and a capacity for the body to improve and get stronger while under fatigue. It is similar to a repetition maximum with lifting weights: in order to gain, the client needs to push it, but not at the expense of good technique.

Power-Based Exercise Example: Maximal Medicine Ball Slam

When programming, it is important to use both endurance-based and power-based exercises. As a tonic muscle, the core requires on-going activation during day-to-day activities, but the body also requires power qualities. These will be relevant to sporting populations, for whom explosive movement patterns may be necessary, powered from the lumbo-pelvic hip region and sling systems. Medicine ball throws, wood chops and band or cable work can all be used to work on explosivity. As with any strength programme, the sets and repetitions for power-based exercises will be different from those for the endurance-based/activation exercises.

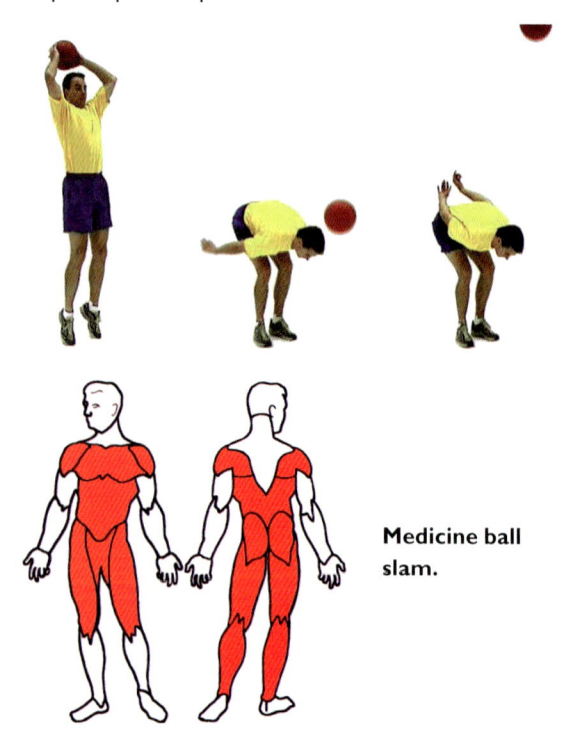

The maximal medicine ball slam is one example of a power-based exercise, which can be progressed as required by making changes to the sets, repetitions, tempo and load.

Sport-specific relevance: an excellent athletic movement pattern can be developed via triple flexion at the start position (ankles, knees and hips), extending up to full triple extension (ankles, knees and hips) and then returning in a coordinated manner to flexion in order to slam the medicine ball into the ground. The medicine ball is then retrieved and the movements repeated. The posterior chain and core-pelvic and glute region must work hard to control the movements and create an integrated force production as the slam is coordinated. Depending on the sets and repetitions, which can be manipulated, a good heart rate response can also be elicited. It requires good core strength and capacity as well as whole-body coordination.

Specific sports that would benefit: multi-directional sports, rugby union, rugby league, ice hockey, field hockey, basketball, track and field, particularly throws and jumps (javelin, shot, high jump and long jump), boxing, wrestling and martial arts. Medicine ball slams are good general athletic power-based exercises, which can benefit most athletic disciplines.

As with any programme, the prescription – the sets, repetitions, load, rest, frequency, tempo, intensity and progressions – for both endurance-based core exercises (such as the plank hold) and power-based core exercises (such as the maximal medicine ball slam) needs to be established. The S&C practitioner must be considerate of any injury history or contraindication for each exercise prescribed, in addition to the individual's competence

Medicine ball slam.

Maximal Medicine Ball Slam

Maximal medicine ball slam	Sets and rest	Reps	Tempo	Frequency	Load	Progression
Level 1: Introductory	2–3 sets 2–3 minutes	4–5 repetitions	Explosive	2–3 × each week	Medicine ball: load determined by capacity for quick power-based movement. Usually around 4–8kg to begin with for a beginner but depending on the individual.	Speed of movement maintained – medicine ball load increased. Excellent technique
Level 2: Body awareness developed – good strength progressions	3–4 sets 2–5 minutes	5 repetitions	Explosive	2–3 × each week	As the individual becomes more efficient the medicine ball load can increase but it is important that the speed of movement is maintained (quick/power-based movement).	Speed of movement/medicine ball load increased. Can introduce single-leg stance or throw and sprint or throw and jump for example.
Level 3: Body awareness is excellent, and strength and power/explosivity is developing well	4–5 sets 2–5 minutes	5 repetitions Can super set with additional exercises, for example: dead lift or clean or drop jumps/counter movement jump, for example (other power-based exercises)	Explosive movement maintained	2–3 × each week	As the individual becomes stronger the medicine ball load can increase but it is important that the speed of movement is maintained (quick/power-based movement).	Speed of movement/medicine ball load increased. Can introduce eccentric involvement: throw and catch or extension/flexion/rotations through range for the start of the slam. Side slam against wall, rotational floor slam and catch, etc.
Level 4 and on-going	Consider on-going progressions but ensure quality movement patterns throughout. It is likely that the level achieved by dedicated work at this point will continue to be stimulated by the activities and external load progressions prescribed at Level 3. Variations can be introduced to include manipulation of sets and reps and the weight of the medicine ball. Focus still on explosivity and the development of power.					

APPLIED CORE CONDITIONING: PROGRAMMING, PRESCRIPTION

NSCA RESISTANCE TRAINING GUIDELINES

The National Strength and Conditioning Association provides the following table in its *Essentials of Strength Training and Conditioning* (2000), as a guideline in exercise prescription based upon training goals.

Training goal	Number of sets	Number of repetitions	Rest between sets
Muscular endurance	3–4	12–15 RM	30–60 seconds
Muscular hypertrophy	3–5	8–12 RM	60–90 seconds
Strength	3–5	Heavy resistance < 6 RM	> 2 minutes
Power	3–5	1–5 RM	> 2 minutes

For the power-based medicine ball slam, an effective exercise prescription would mirror what is advised above with appropriate sets and repetition options. For muscular endurance and strength development, the prescription may be repetition-based or also based upon duration, as with the plank hold.

THE FORCE–VELOCITY CURVE

The force–velocity curve needs to be considered when selecting load and considering target outcomes for the individual. If the load is too heavy, the movement will become slow and more strength-based; if it is too light, it will become more speed-based. The exercise needs to be executed with the correct loading demands to ensure power development and explosivity, if these are the target outcomes, as with the medicine ball slam.

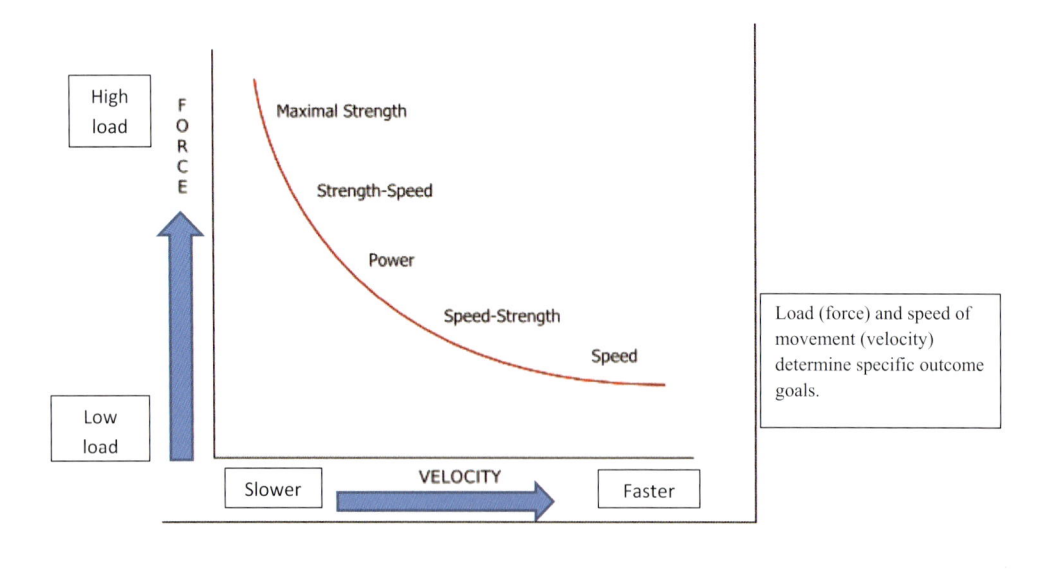

Load (force) and speed of movement (velocity) determine specific outcome goals.

and ability to perform each exercise well, ensuring correct form. Each set must always be performed with excellent technique, despite some appropriate muscular overload to ensure adaptation and progress. Progression of the exercises is always directed by the competency of the individual. If competency is poor, there is no progression.

SPORTS-SPECIFIC CONDITIONING AND PROGRAMME DESIGN

As the core behaves in a state of constant tonic activation, with Type I fibres activating – slow-contracting, high resistance to fatigue with a low force production – it makes sense generally to train this way for this group of muscles. Only when higher, more power-based demands are placed upon the area would the Type IIA and Type IIB fibres kick in. These muscle fibre types are less resistant to fatigue. The goals of the individual will determine what type of core exercises are prescribed: static/isometric repetition-based/duration-based, which are more resistant to fatigue, or more explosive, power-based exercises. The latter may create more power development but an individual's capacity to complete a large number or for a long duration is limited, as the relevant muscle fibre types are less resistant to fatigue. This training option would be very sport-specific – relevant for a tennis player or boxer, for example, who requires power and strength. There are differences in exercise selection and programming decisions when dealing with a sedentary individual with low back pain, for example, and a tennis player who wants to improve performance. Specificity of training and the individual's requirements, goals and history are all key to appropriate and successful programming and prescription.

There is of course a point at which a good foundation of core strength, muscle activation and lumbar-pelvic control has been achieved, when it is possible to be more prescriptive according to the specific requirements and demands of the sport or activity in which the individual is involved. It is possible to be more creative with the demands placed upon the core and associated musculature, and consider the more functional demands placed upon the body, depending on the sport completed. There is of course a crossover into all sports and physical activity with strengthening the core, but it is possible to fine-tune the movement pattern to mimic the loading required in a particular sport. Equally, it is relevant to consider the physical demands placed upon the body and how a strong and well-conditioned core, lumbo-pelvic region and posterior chain can have a positive outcome on performance, as well as on robustness and injury prevention.

Many of the sports and disciplines covered may have similar physiological demands. For example, field hockey can be classified as a rotation sport because of the mechanism of rotation with the hockey stick held in a flexed position, yet is also a high-intensity intermittent sport, which requires additional high-quality physical preparation. Players need to be physically prepared to cope with the multifaceted demands placed upon their body and their core. Rowing is another example – an endurance sport but performed while seated, with repetitive high loading. Many athletes will have a complete strength and conditioning programme provided and prescribed, and also a dedicated core programme to complement the more compound, performance-based exercises. On many occasions, the exercise completed will challenge both the core musculature as well as benefit performance outcomes.

Athletes at both the recreational level and the highest level need to be able to control acceleration and deceleration, concentric and eccentric demands, multi-directional movements and reactive forces, as well as manage contact with other athletes and be resilient to force placed upon the body. It is essential that the core and associated musculature, including the lumbo-pelvic region, posterior chain and sling systems, are conditioned to cope with these demands, otherwise it is likely that injury will occur.

In physical development, form follows function, so it is very likely that playing tennis, squash or basketball, or rowing, for example, will lead to some functional core development as a result of a particular movement pattern and the frequency of loading, irrespective of any specific core conditioning programme. However, in order to accelerate performance and reduce injury potential, the athlete will need to create a more robust and resilient body. This is done by following an effective, specific core conditioning programme, which may include isolated exercises as well as multi-planar and compound exercises.

Based upon the movement patterns, the physical stressors and the demands of different sports, four key sporting categories have been identified below. Examples are also given of how to train and improve core conditioning relevant to these specific sporting challenges and requirements. Some exercises are of course beneficial for all sports, but the exercise options below have been selected to condition the demands of that key component and category, to improve function, resilience, performance and robustness. The list of sports is not exhaustive but provides an indication of what movement patterns to consider when planning and designing a core strengthening programme centred around the physical demands of the sport. The four main categories are:

1. **Rotation sports**: tennis, badminton, squash, golf, discus, javelin, cricket, baseball, softball, hockey, ice hockey, martial arts, judo, boxing, kayaking, canoeing, water polo, wrestling, lacrosse.
2. **Multi-directional high-intensity intermittent sports**: football/soccer, rugby league, rugby union, basketball, American football, volleyball, hockey, ice hockey, netball, Gaelic football, Australian Rules.
3. **Seated events**: horse riding, motor racing, motorbike speedway, cycling, BMX, bobsleigh, rowing, kayak, canoeing.
4. **Endurance and linear events**: running, triathlon, athletics, Nordic skiing, rowing, archery, skiing, fencing, gymnastics, sailing, triathlon, speed skating, swimming, hurdles.

Rotation Sports

Tennis, badminton, squash, golf, discus, javelin, cricket, baseball, softball, field hockey, ice hockey, martial arts, judo, boxing, kayaking, canoeing, water polo, wrestling, lacrosse.

Once a level of foundation strength and control has been reached, then it makes sense to include specific rotational movements that demand both concentric and eccentric force. These will evolve to become more explosive due to the nature and demands of these particular sports. This is where the serape effect and the sling systems will be put to use within the body's musculature. Selecting whole-body exercises, such as lunge patterns, wood chops, cable rotations, and so on, will all be very functional. If the athlete is seated, as in a kayak or canoe, then seated cable work, medicine ball work or band work will also be very functional.

The following selection of rotational movement patterns are aimed at specifically conditioning the core and associated musculature to help with protection, robustness and performance in rotation sports. There are also a number of examples of specific rotational sports that would benefit from the particular movement patterns. Paying heed to the stance – whether the athlete is seated or standing in a split stance as they rotate, whether they are rotating through a full range of movement or partial, left- or right-sided only or both sides – will add to the specificity of movement.

The selected exercise examples demonstrate how varied the training modality can be for rotation sports. Using external equipment; varying the grip on a band or cable; working single-leg stance or double-leg stance, or wide or split stance; working seated or standing or kneeling; all will affect the demands of the exercise and can ensure specificity to the desired sport and outcome.

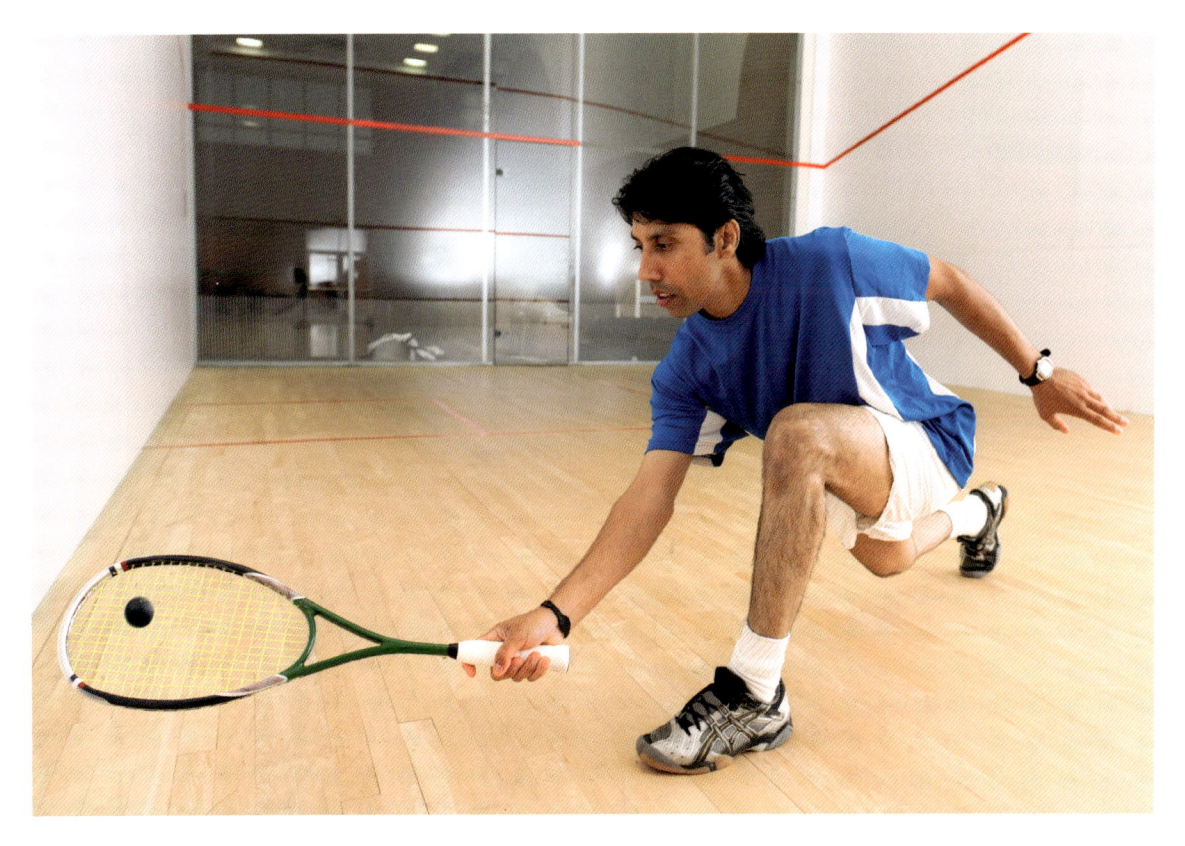

APPLIED CORE CONDITIONING: PROGRAMMING, PRESCRIPTION

A squash player requires good agility, lower body strength and explosive power through the core musculature to perform well, with quickness, explosivity and a deft touch.

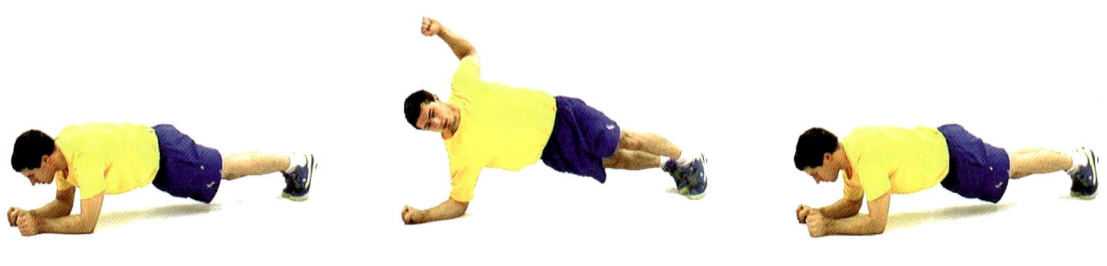

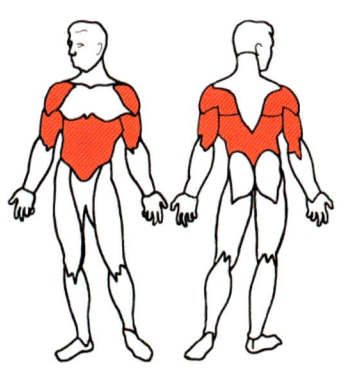

Stabilization rotation: progression of a foundation plank hold exercise.

Many of these exercise options presented here can not only be applied to any rotational sport, but can also become part of an evolving programme for other sports. For example, the tyre rotation is a fun and demanding exercise that a rugby player may enjoy. In their sport, they have rotational demands placed upon them, with passing and kicking the ball, as well as multi-directional demands. Crossing some of the options over into other sports can make the programme design more exciting and varied. As the

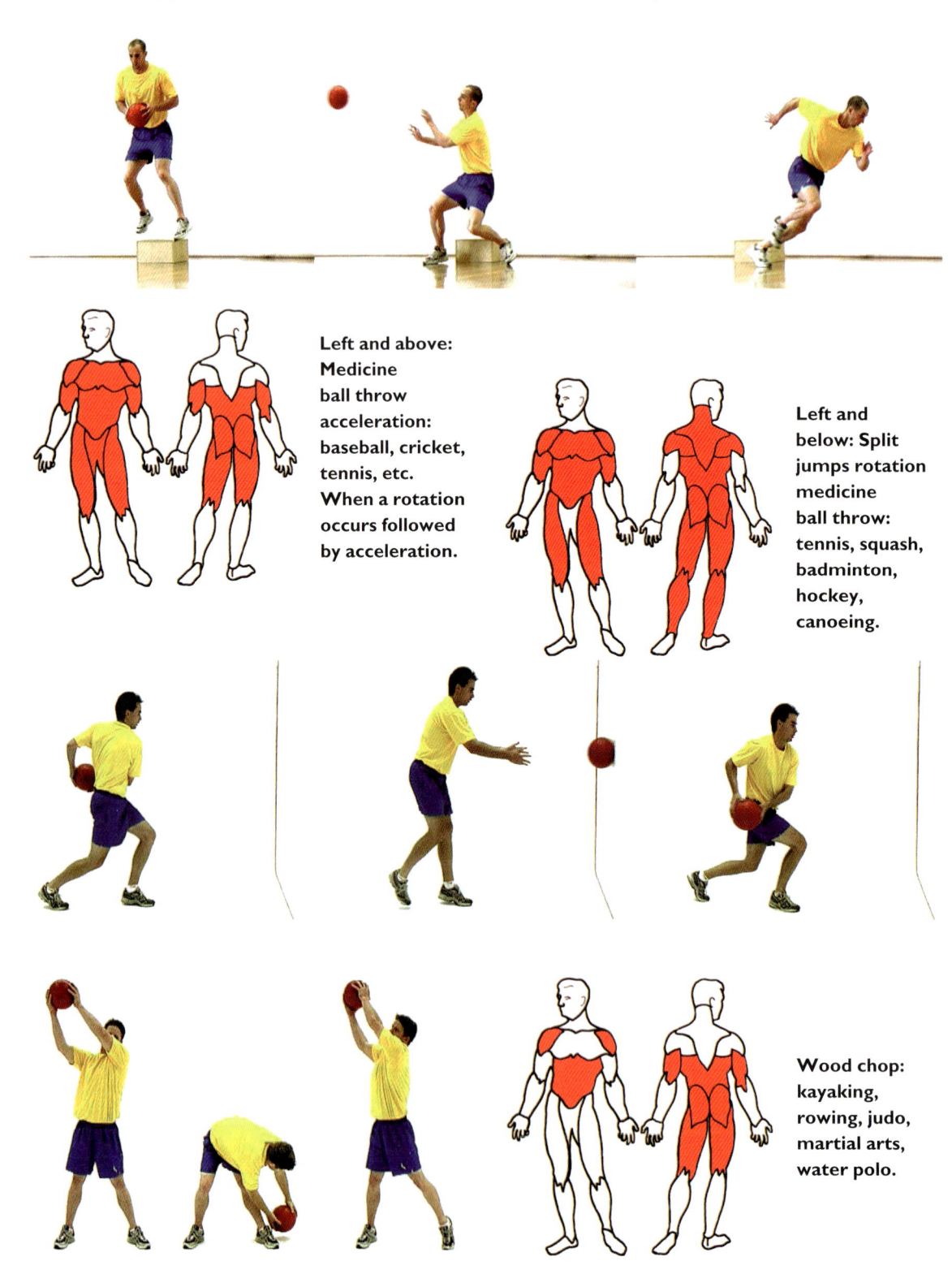

APPLIED CORE CONDITIONING: PROGRAMMING, PRESCRIPTION

Left and above: Medicine ball throw acceleration: baseball, cricket, tennis, etc. When a rotation occurs followed by acceleration.

Left and below: Split jumps rotation medicine ball throw: tennis, squash, badminton, hockey, canoeing.

Wood chop: kayaking, rowing, judo, martial arts, water polo.

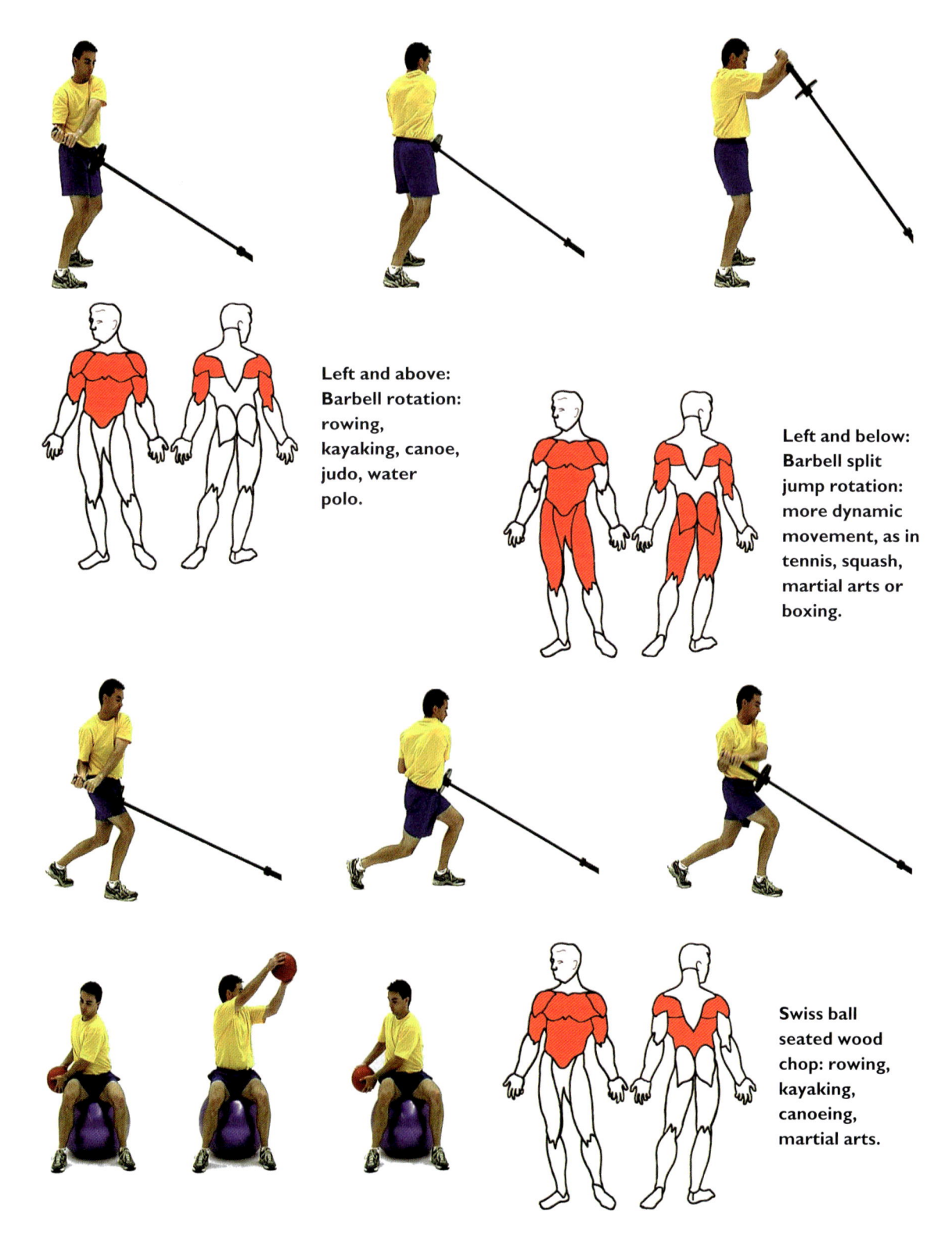

APPLIED CORE CONDITIONING: PROGRAMMING, PRESCRIPTION

Left and above: Barbell rotation: rowing, kayaking, canoe, judo, water polo.

Left and below: Barbell split jump rotation: more dynamic movement, as in tennis, squash, martial arts or boxing.

Swiss ball seated wood chop: rowing, kayaking, canoeing, martial arts.

127

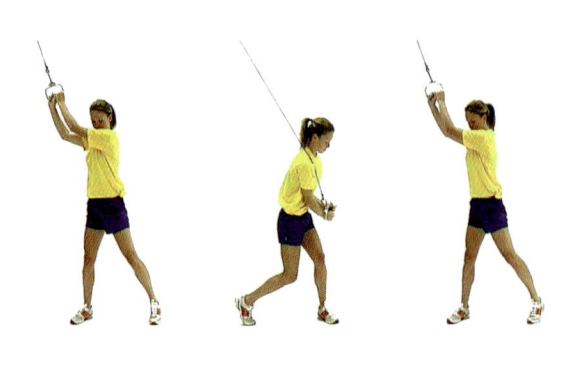

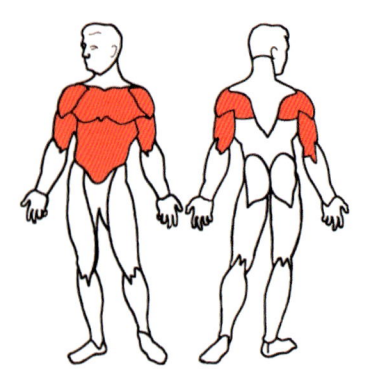

APPLIED CORE CONDITIONING: PROGRAMMING, PRESCRIPTION

Cable rotation: golf, cricket, hockey (ice and field), lacrosse.

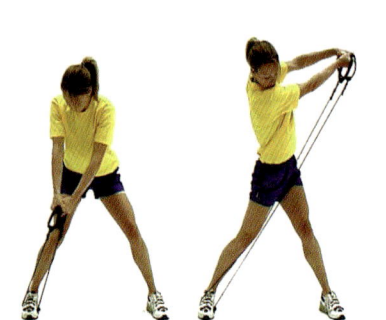

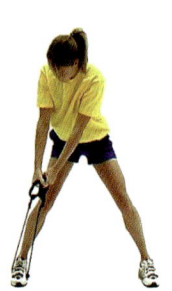

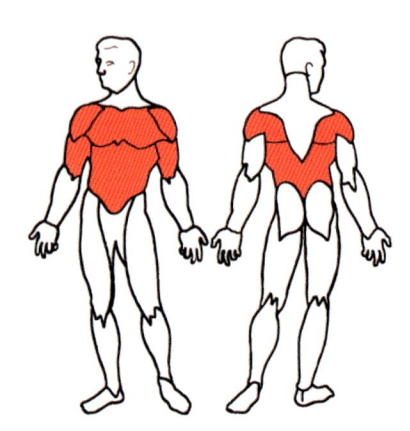

Band rotation: golf, cricket, baseball, softball, hockey (ice and field), lacrosse.

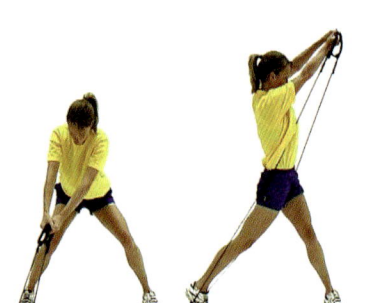

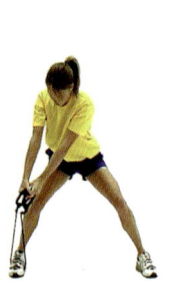

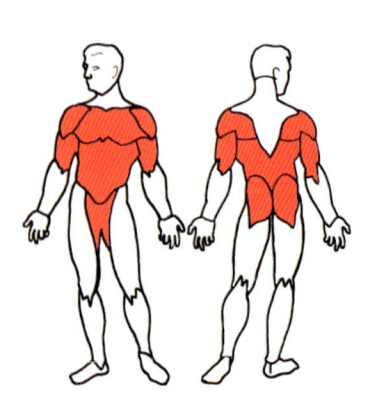

Band rotation: hockey-specific. Wider stance relates to baseball or softball.

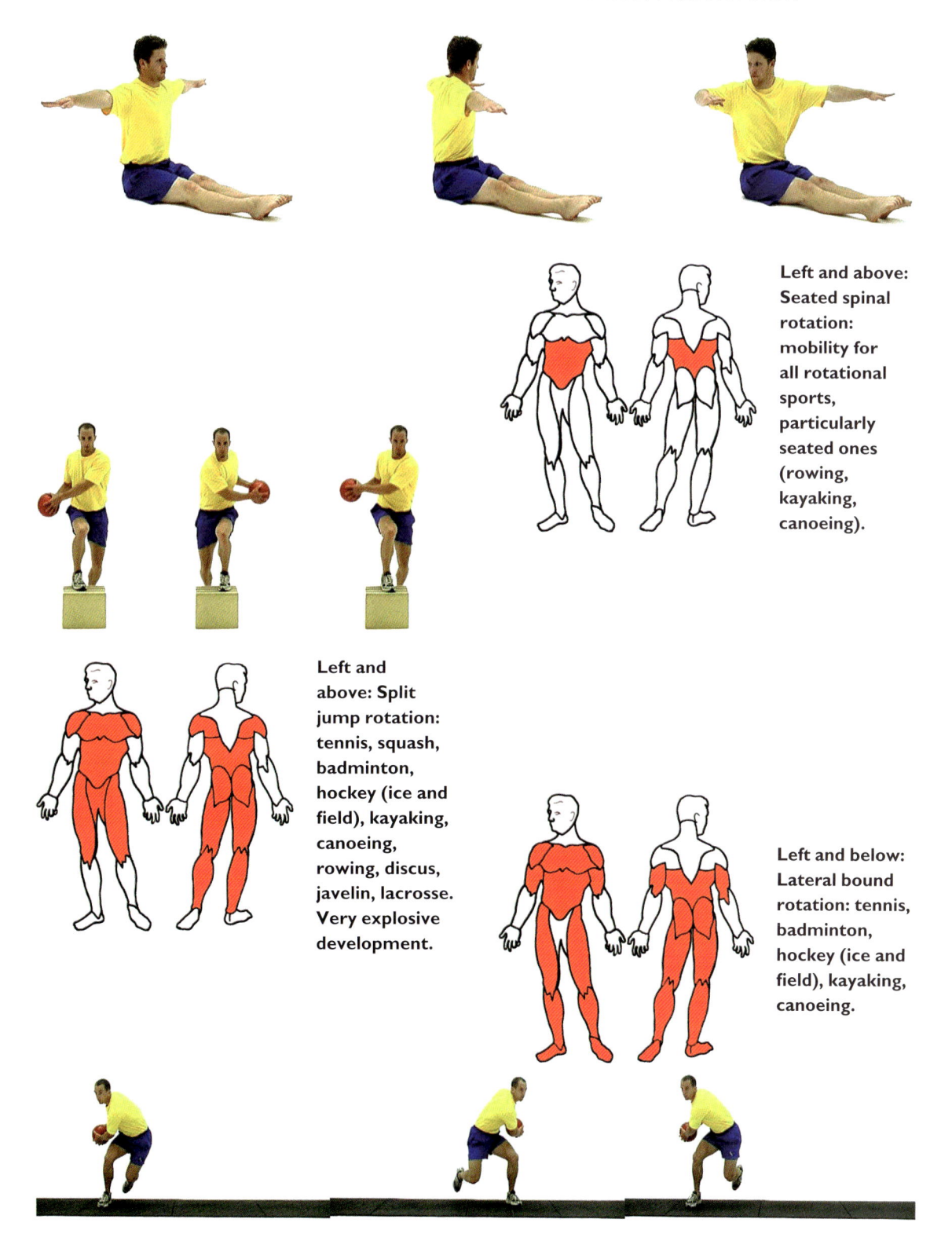

APPLIED CORE CONDITIONING: PROGRAMMING, PRESCRIPTION

Left and above: Seated spinal rotation: mobility for all rotational sports, particularly seated ones (rowing, kayaking, canoeing).

Left and above: Split jump rotation: tennis, squash, badminton, hockey (ice and field), kayaking, canoeing, rowing, discus, javelin, lacrosse. Very explosive development.

Left and below: Lateral bound rotation: tennis, badminton, hockey (ice and field), kayaking, canoeing.

129

APPLIED CORE CONDITIONING: PROGRAMMING, PRESCRIPTION

Left and above: Single-leg cable rotation: tennis, badminton, squash, hockey (field and ice), martial arts.

Left and below: Cable rotation: canoeing, kayaking, martial arts.

BOSU medicine ball throw: tennis, squash, badminton, cricket, hockey (ice and field), baseball, softball.

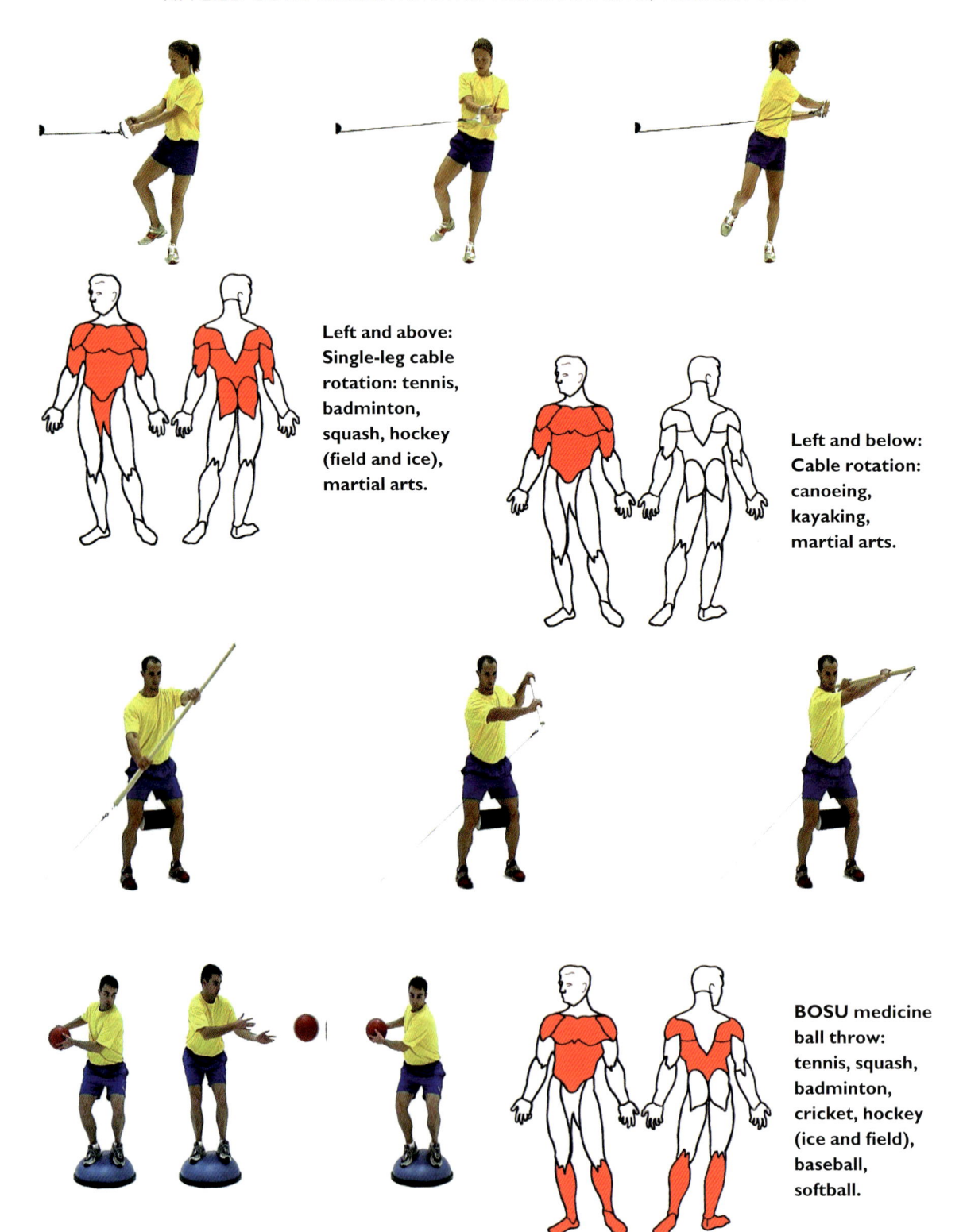

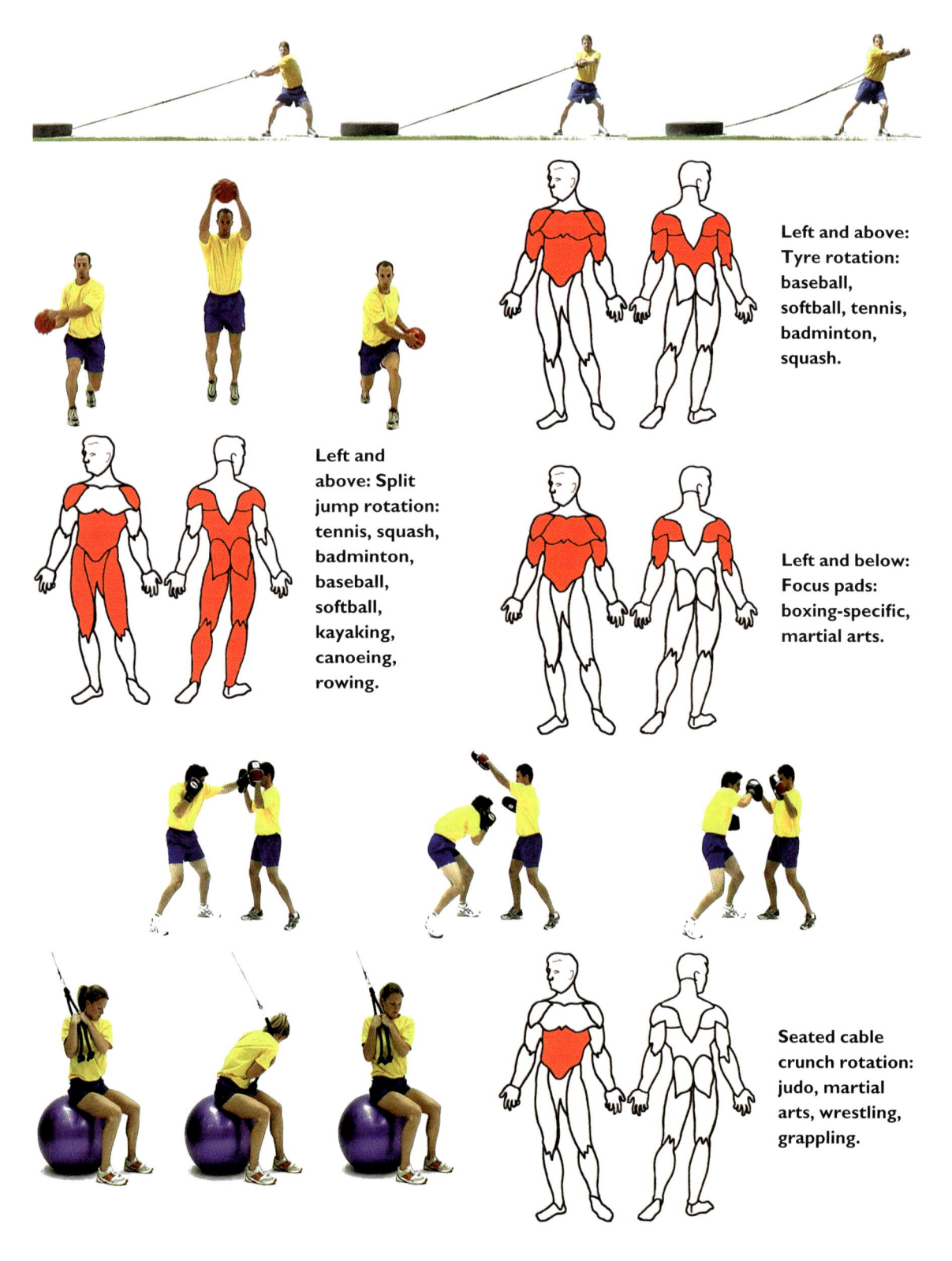

APPLIED CORE CONDITIONING: PROGRAMMING, PRESCRIPTION

Left and above: Tyre rotation: baseball, softball, tennis, badminton, squash.

Left and above: Split jump rotation: tennis, squash, badminton, baseball, softball, kayaking, canoeing, rowing.

Left and below: Focus pads: boxing-specific, martial arts.

Seated cable crunch rotation: judo, martial arts, wrestling, grappling.

131

APPLIED CORE CONDITIONING: PROGRAMMING, PRESCRIPTION

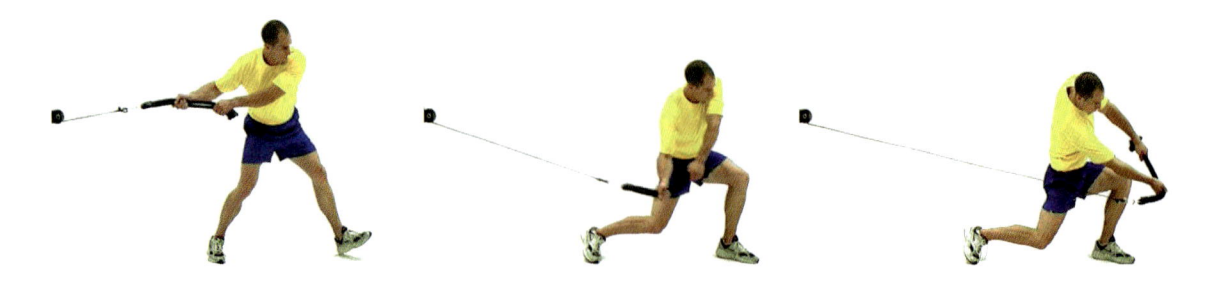

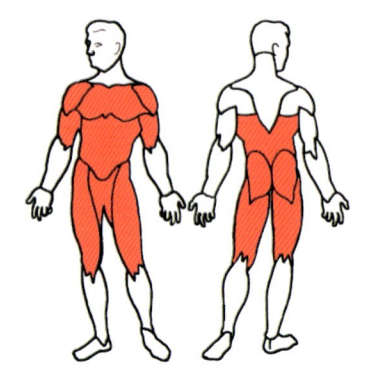

Cable rotation: cricket, hockey (ice and field), baseball, softball, lacrosse.

This would evolve from more simple movement patterns, using a cable or band, to a whole-body challenge, with a sprint or lower limb split squat being performed with a medicine ball rotation or medicine ball throw. These can be highly demanding and complex movement patterns, but they are valuable for well-conditioned athletes in high-performance sports.

conditioning programme evolves, creativity can add to the fun and make it more challenging, as well as specific and relevant.

Exercise selection: isometric holds progress to more dynamic rotation-based movement patterns.

Multi-Directional High-Intensity Intermittent Sports

Football/soccer, rugby league, rugby union, basketball, American football, volleyball, field hockey, ice hockey, netball, Gaelic football, Australian Rules.

Programme design and prescription for core conditioning for rotational sports

Sets	Repetitions	Tempo	Load	Frequency
3–5 sets	5–12 repetitions	Variable depending on the outcome goals: explosive or focus on eccentric loading or concentric loading, for example: 2-0-2 4-1-2 2-1-4 2-4-2 1-1-2	Progressive but must lead to an overload/repetition maximum on the exercises. Consider the force–velocity curve for optimal loading in relation to targets. Always performed with quality.	3–4 x each week 3–4 exercises selected depending on phase of training within compound strength programme. Dedicated core strength conditioning is necessary for the rotational demands of these sports.

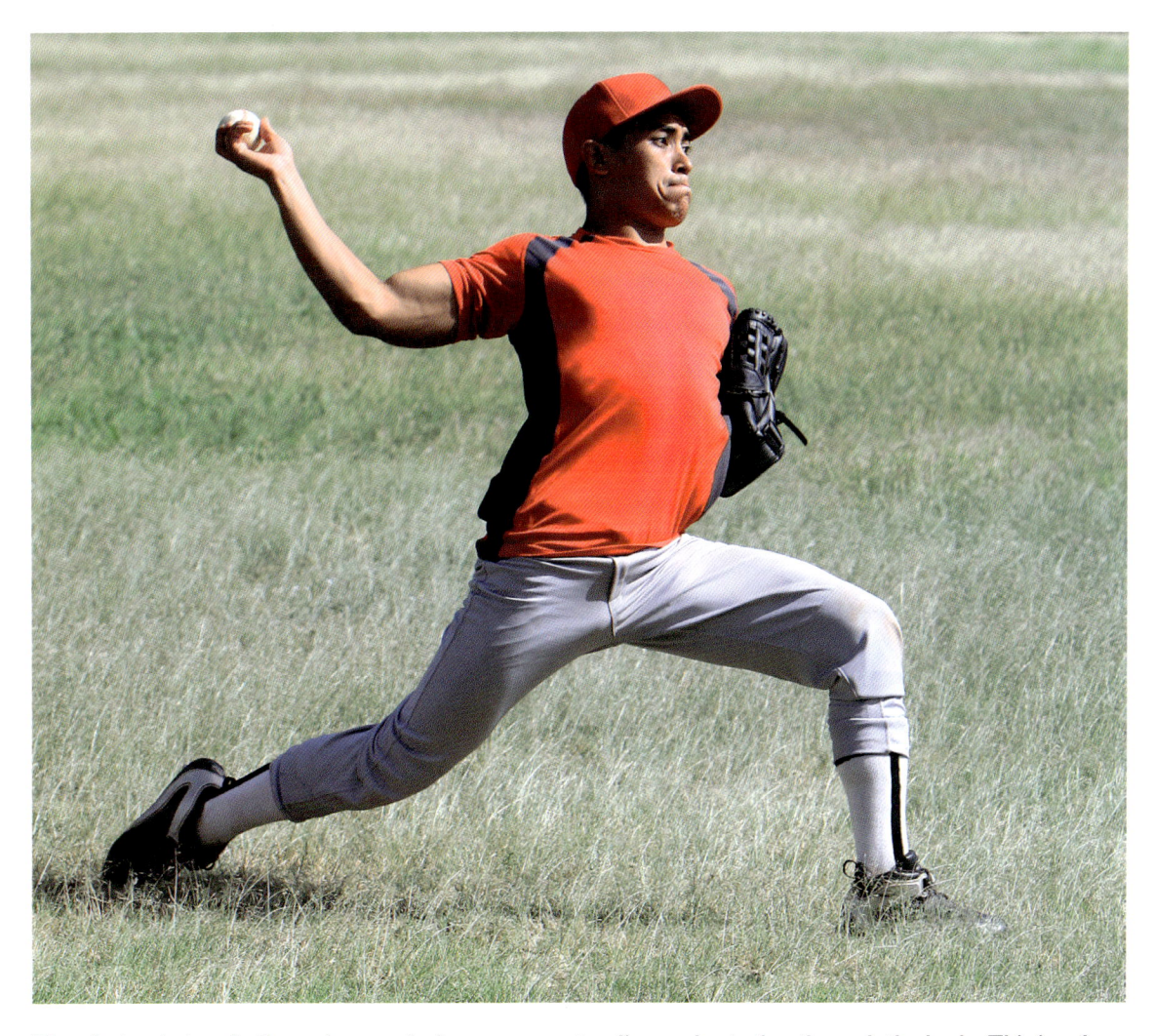

APPLIED CORE CONDITIONING: PROGRAMMING, PRESCRIPTION

The pitcher in baseball requires explosive power, extending and rotating through the body. This involves whole-body coordination and a link through the posterior chain, core and lumbo-thoracic region. It is a great example of the sling systems at work.

The demands of high-intensity intermittent sports on the body are significant. The risk of injury is increased due to the repeated contact with other athletes, and injuries such as hamstring tears and ankle sprains are common. Hawkins *et al.* (2001) completed a prospective epidemiological study of the injuries sustained in English professional football over two competitive seasons. Player injuries were annotated by club medical staff at 91 professional football clubs. A specific injury audit questionnaire was used, together with a weekly form that documented each club's current injury status. They established that pre-season injuries were more prevalent than in-season injuries, indicating that the players are not conditioned appropriately to cope with the early physical demands placed upon them.

The distribution of injury was as follows: strains (37 per cent) and sprains (19 per cent) were the major injury types, with the lower extremity being the site of 87 per cent of the injuries reported. Most injury mechanisms were classified as being non-contact (58 per cent). Re-injuries accounted for 7 per cent of all injuries (Hawkins et al., 2001). The fact that the incidence of non-contact injuries was high indicates that conditioning was perhaps not optimal, which placed the players at risk. The research suggested that there was an average of 1.3 injuries per player per season. The mean (SD) number of days absent for each injury was 24.2 (40.2), with 78 per cent of the injuries leading to a minimum of one competitive match being missed (Hawkins et al., 2001) – potentially very costly for a team. Professional football has changed a lot since 2001, with more S&C staffing, physiotherapists, physiologists, nutrition support and better-educated management and coaches, which should all lead to better knowledge and less incidence of non-contact injury.

Functional conditioning, with high-end applied activities, is important for footballers, as it is for players of any multi-directional sport: basketball, field hockey, volleyball and rugby, for example. A good foundation needs to be introduced and maintained with the youth and academy players, then developed with the young professionals and into the first team squad. It is very important to have a strong posterior chain, to cope with acceleration and deceleration activities. A strong core will support the groin, hip flexors and lumbar spine, which all have significant demands placed upon them, with high-intensity multi-directional movements and the kicking in football, Australian Rules and rugby. Injury prevention in these sports is smart and cost-effective, allowing a healthy, uninjured squad of players to be available for selection week in, week out. As the demands placed upon the body include whole-body movements – aerobic and anaerobic actions, and multi-directional reactive and contact forces, to name but a few – once a foundation of strength and core capacity has been achieved, it is possible to become very functional in the exercise selection. There would certainly be some benefit in combining more isolated core-strengthening exercises in addition to whole-body movement patterns.

As an example, a volleyball player moves, steps, jumps and spikes in a restricted area. Their movement patterns include triple flexion and triple extension, with squatting and dipping and then extending to spike the ball. They draw on their capacity for endurance as well as power. They also need good mobility, to get around the court and flex into low positions to defend and pass the ball, in addition to an ability to extend powerfully and smash a spike when required.

How can a volleyball player train and condition for these complex demands? What is the best way to prevent low back pain or hamstring problems in such a demanding sport? In my view, volleyball, as well as probably all the multi-directional sports that involve acceleration and deceleration and flexion and extension, demands a strong core foundation. This is achieved by carrying on early-stage isometric work and then moving on to strengthening the posterior chain, working on cables and bands and with medicine balls for extension and flexion, similar to the athletes from the rotational sports. When the extremities are moving a cable or band, or a dumbbell or barbell, the individual is involved in multi-planar movement patterns. The lower limbs are included as part of this core conditioning, using lunge patterns, Olympic lifts, compound exercises and balance work. Cables are used to complete adduction/abduction while bracing through the core. Challenging single-leg stance positions are valuable, as this is a position that a volleyball player (or other sportsperson) is likely to be in if or when contact occurs. Again, the S&C coach can be creative in coming up with a programme, but always considering the specific demands of the sport.

A progression to more dynamic whole-body exercises within the selection above is recommended, considering the physical and metabolic demands placed upon this type of athlete. There should be a transition from the foundation core exercises into more applied, functional movement

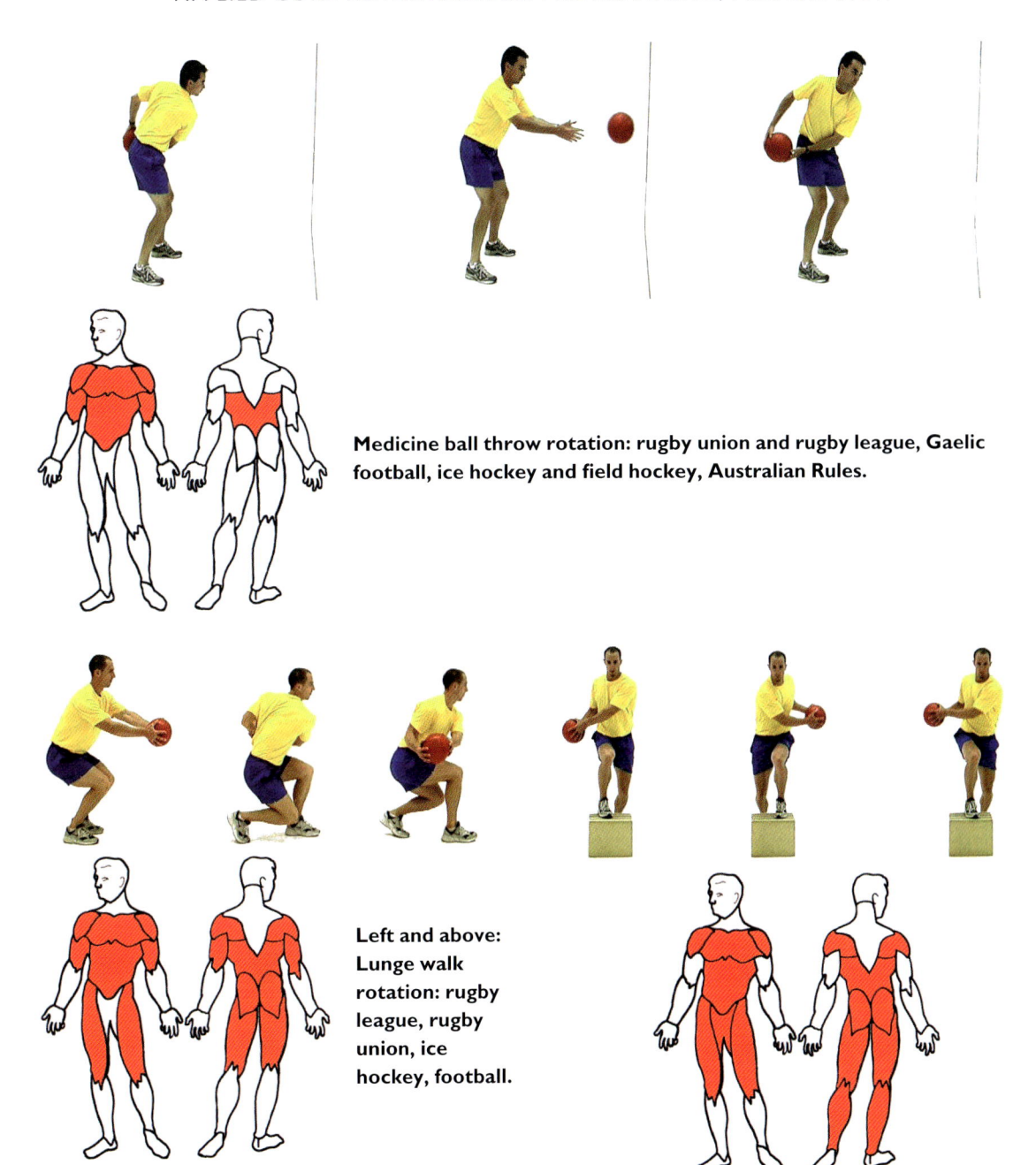

APPLIED CORE CONDITIONING: PROGRAMMING, PRESCRIPTION

Medicine ball throw rotation: rugby union and rugby league, Gaelic football, ice hockey and field hockey, Australian Rules.

Left and above: Lunge walk rotation: rugby league, rugby union, ice hockey, football.

Above: Split jumps rotation: football/soccer, rugby league, rugby union, basketball, American football, volleyball, field hockey, ice hockey, netball, Gaelic football, Australian Rules.

135

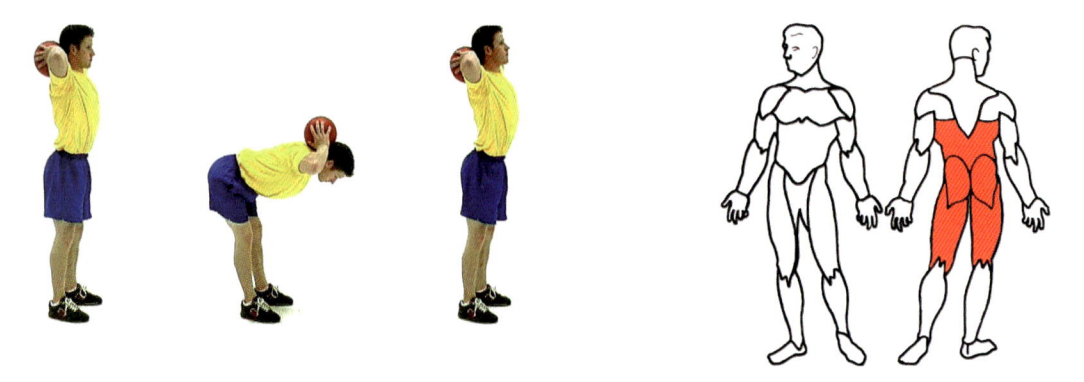

APPLIED CORE CONDITIONING: PROGRAMMING, PRESCRIPTION

Medicine ball good morning, for strengthening the posterior chain: football, rugby league, rugby union, basketball, American football, volleyball, field hockey, ice hockey, netball, Gaelic football, Australian Rules.

Swiss ball roll out stabilization (progression from foundation plank hold): football, rugby league, rugby union, basketball, American football, volleyball, field hockey, ice hockey, netball, Gaelic football, Australian Rules.

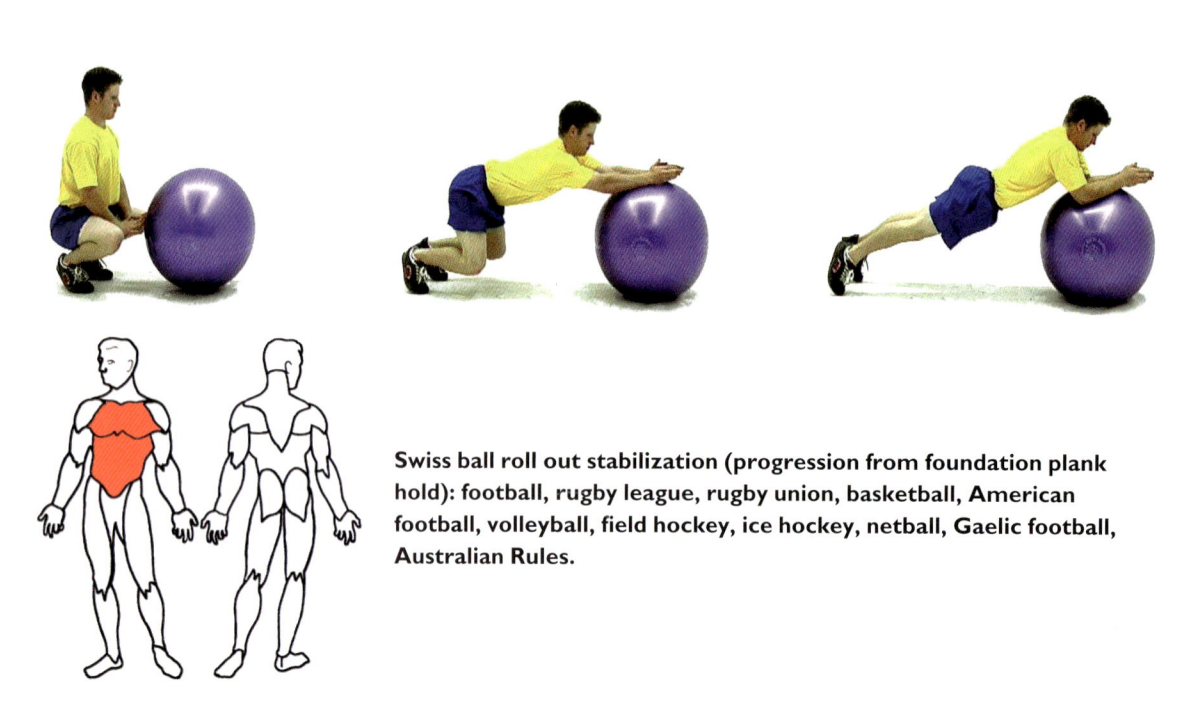

patterns, which challenge the whole body, but the early stage exercises must be completed, and the athlete must be competent, before progressing.

The benefits of the compound lifts in a programme are that the core and trunk musculature will be conditioned and challenged, and that there should also be performance gains from completing these exercises.

The exercises included place whole-body demands on the athlete, to help prepare them for high-intensity multi-directional activity. There is a focus on the posterior chain, as the demands of acceleration and deceleration and change of direction are high, and these athletes need to be able to cope with this through the lumbo-pelvic region as well as having excellent hamstring capacity and strength.

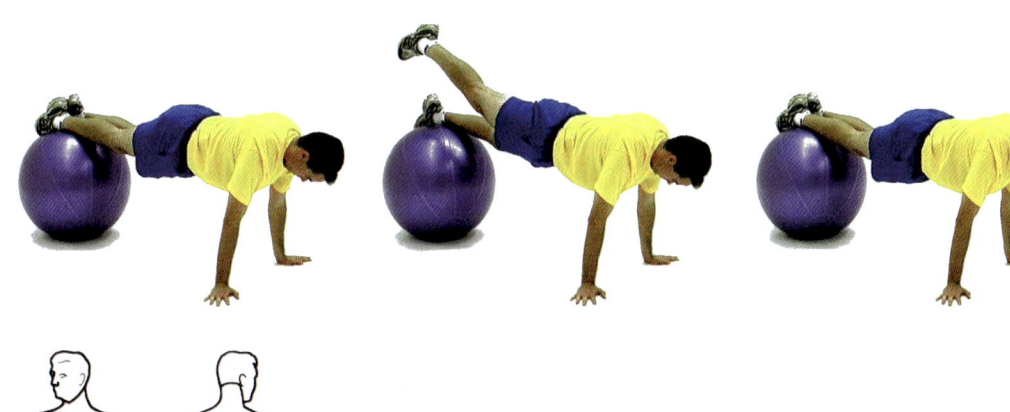

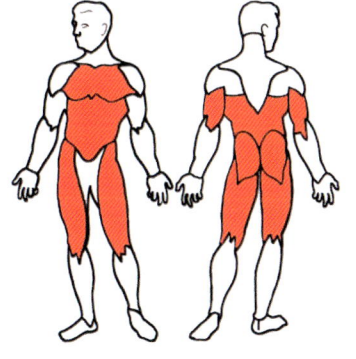

APPLIED CORE CONDITIONING: PROGRAMMING, PRESCRIPTION

Swiss ball hip extension (progression from plank hold), for strengthening the posterior chain: football, rugby league, rugby union, basketball, American football, volleyball, field hockey, ice hockey, netball, Gaelic football, Australian Rules.

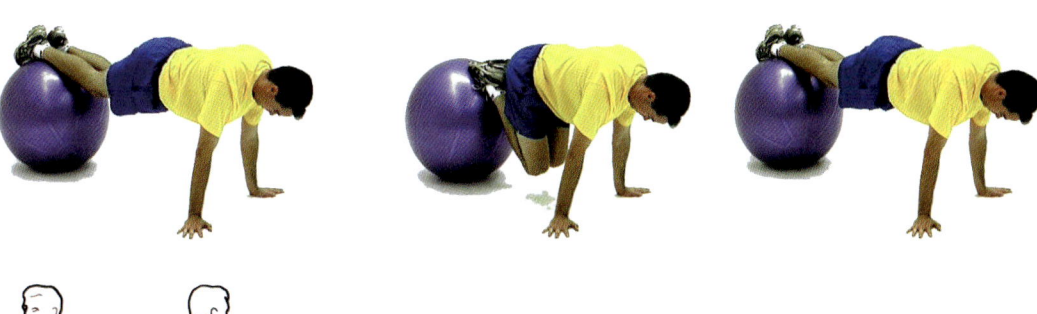

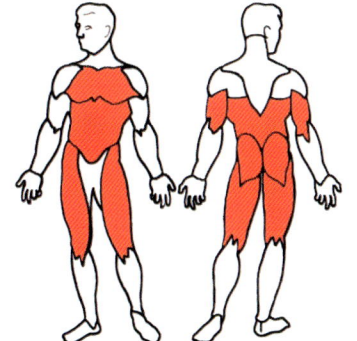

Swiss ball hip flexion, for the posterior chain, core and hip flexors. Good for general core conditioning for football/soccer, rugby league, rugby union, basketball, American football, volleyball, field hockey, ice hockey, netball, Gaelic football, Australian Rules.

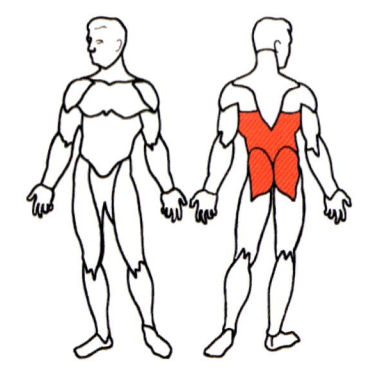

APPLIED CORE CONDITIONING: PROGRAMMING, PRESCRIPTION

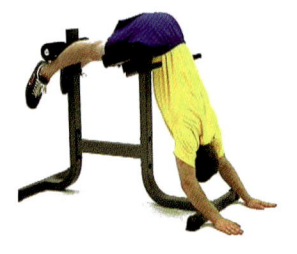

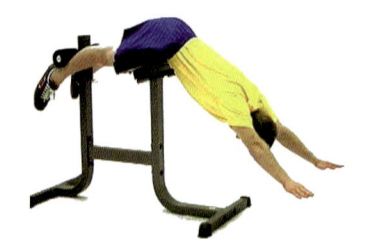

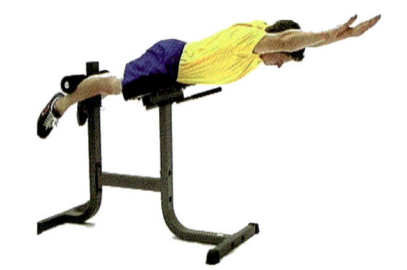

Roman chair back extension, for strengthening the posterior chain: football, rugby league, rugby union, basketball, American football, volleyball, field hockey, ice hockey, netball, Gaelic football, Australian Rules.

The multi-directional sports require a great capacity to complete varied movement patterns with strength and control, but they also often ask the player to be dexterous with the feet or hands. It is therefore important for the conditioning programme to evolve and develop from the core exercises. Some of these options may not be perceived to be traditional core exercises, but they will provide a strength and capacity for the athlete to become robust and strong. Recent research has shown that Olympic lifts, integrated exercises and compound, multi-joint, multi-planar lifts activate the core and lumbo-pelvic musculature (Gottschall *et al.*, 2013 and Nuzzo *et al.*, 2008) and are therefore a smart choice in exercise selection, to transfer to performance as well as core strength development.

Exercise selection: many of the exercises selected are whole-body compound exercises that involve triple flexion and extension at the ankle, knee and hip, as well as posterior chain development. This is essential for acceleration/deceleration and multi-directional sports, which have a high physical demand. The basics should not be forgotten, and the athlete should still complete their foundation core strength exercises: the isometric work, progressed to cable, band and Swiss ball work into more complex movements such as the Olympic lifts, which strengthen the core, as well as improving performance and physical development.

The demands placed upon the body, including the function of the core, in high-intensity intermittent sport are high, and the body must have a capacity to cope with this. If there is a deficiency or imbalance, there will be more risk of injury.

The balance between strength, work capacity and mobility is important, and working throughout a full range of movement while placing demands on the core is certainly going to be protective. Specificity of training is important, but consideration should also be given to combining some of the core exercises with some athletic movements, for example, a medicine ball slam and then sprint; a kettle bell

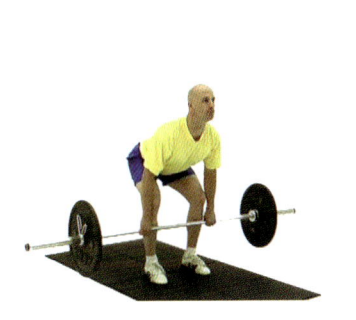

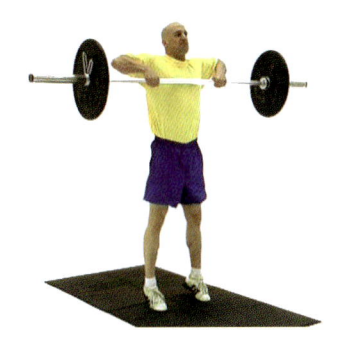

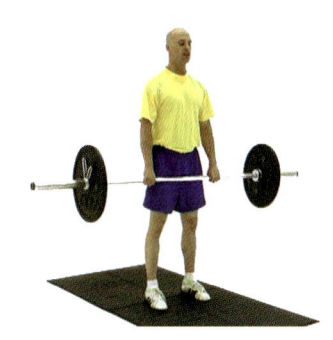

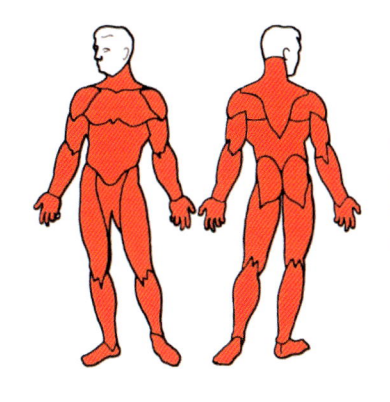

APPLIED CORE CONDITIONING: PROGRAMMING, PRESCRIPTION

Hang clean pull, provides whole-body conditioning with performance benefits: football, rugby league, rugby union, basketball, American football, volleyball, field hockey, ice hockey, netball, Gaelic football, Australian Rules.

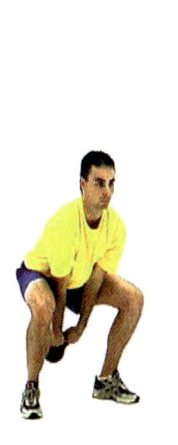

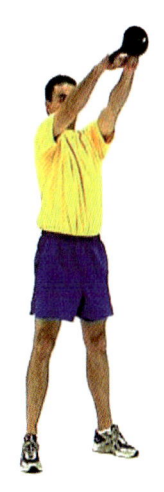

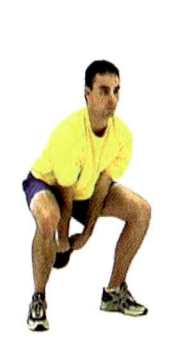

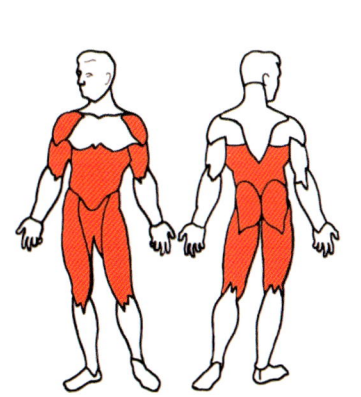

Kettle bell swing, provides whole-body conditioning with performance benefits, and posterior chain development: football, rugby league, rugby union, basketball, American football, volleyball, field hockey, ice hockey, netball, Gaelic football, Australian Rules.

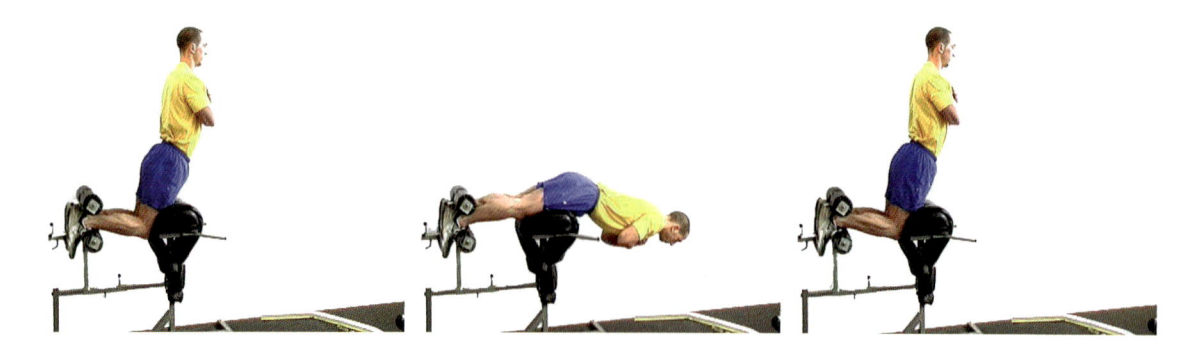

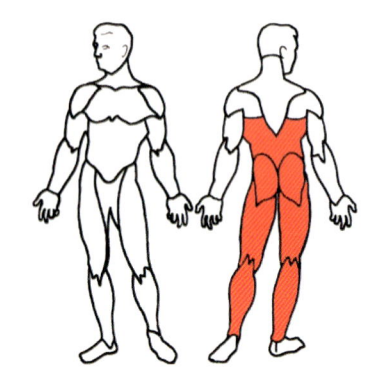

APPLIED CORE CONDITIONING: PROGRAMMING, PRESCRIPTION

Glute-ham-gastroc raise, provides whole-body conditioning with performance benefits, and posterior chain development: football, rugby league, rugby union, basketball, American football, volleyball, field hockey, ice hockey, netball, Gaelic football, Australian Rules.

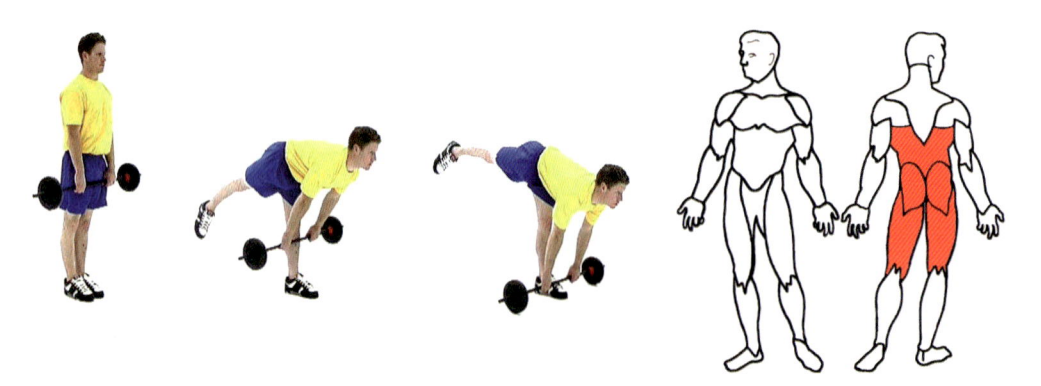

Single-leg straight-leg dead lift (or arabesque), provides posterior chain strength and eccentric load for robustness and injury prevention: football, rugby league, rugby union, basketball, American football, volleyball, field hockey, ice hockey, netball, Gaelic football, Australian Rules.

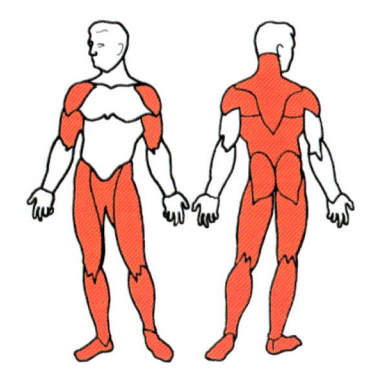

APPLIED CORE CONDITIONING: PROGRAMMING, PRESCRIPTION

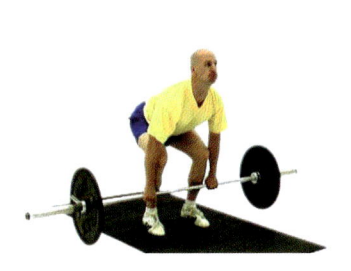

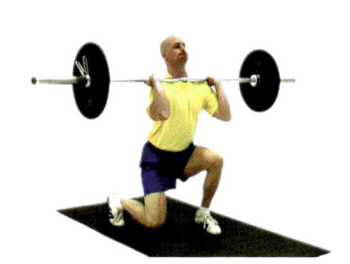

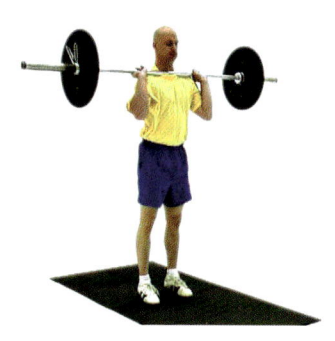

Split clean, provides whole-body conditioning with performance benefits: football, rugby league, rugby union, basketball, American football, volleyball, field hockey, ice hockey, netball, Gaelic football, Australian Rules.

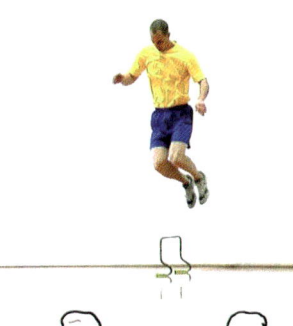

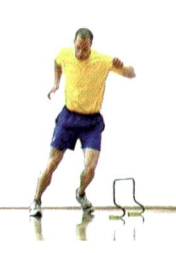

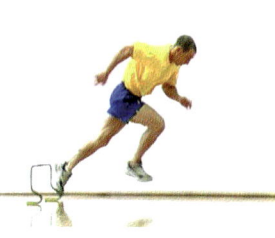

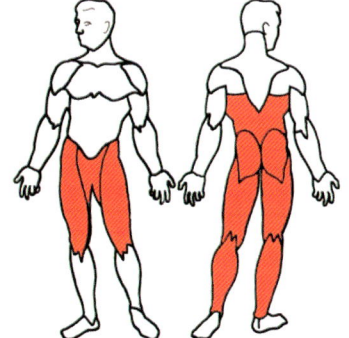

Lateral jump acceleration, provides whole-body conditioning with performance benefits: football, rugby league, rugby union, basketball, American football, volleyball, field hockey, ice hockey, netball, Gaelic football, Australian Rules.

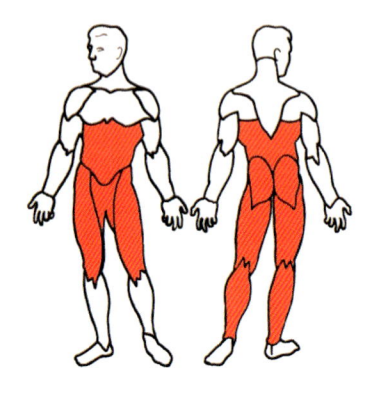

APPLIED CORE CONDITIONING: PROGRAMMING, PRESCRIPTION

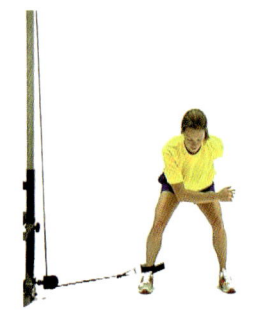

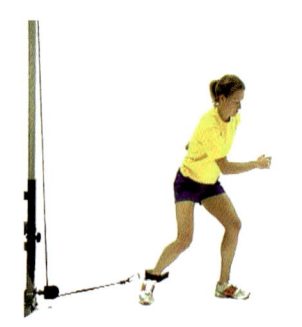

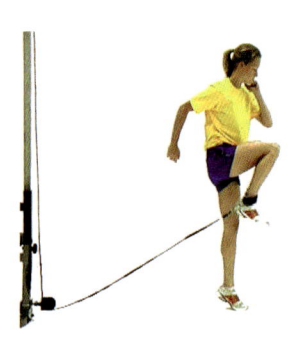

Hip flexion cable extension, provides whole-body conditioning with performance benefits: football, rugby league, rugby union, basketball, American football, volleyball, field hockey, ice hockey, netball, Gaelic football, Australian Rules.

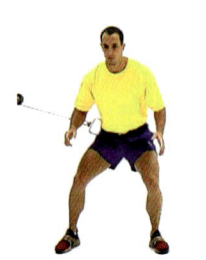

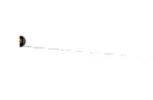

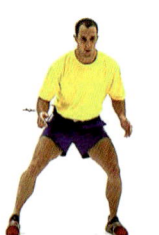

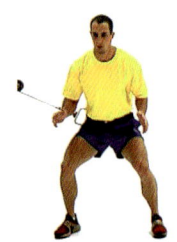

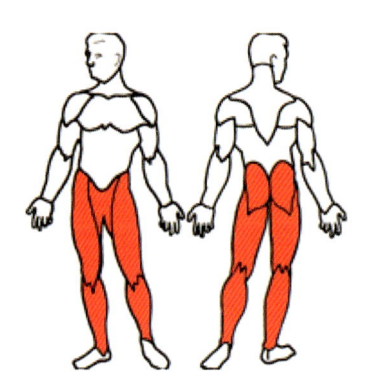

Cable shuffle, provides whole-body conditioning with performance benefits, and posterior chain development: football, rugby league, rugby union, basketball, American football, volleyball, field hockey, ice hockey, netball, Gaelic football, Australian Rules.

APPLIED CORE CONDITIONING: PROGRAMMING, PRESCRIPTION

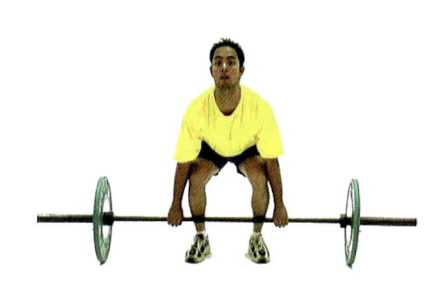

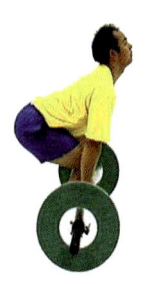

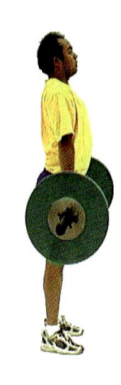

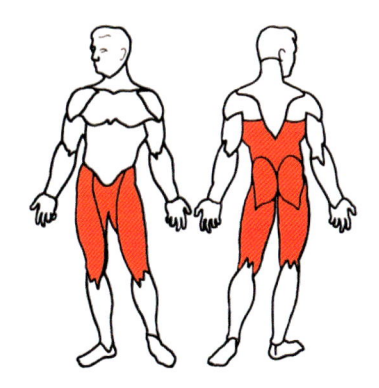

Compound, multi-joint lifts such as the dead lift have been shown to activate the lumbo-pelvic and posterior chain musculature effectively.

Programme design and prescription for core conditioning for high-intensity multi-directional sport

Sets	Repetitions	Tempo	Load	Frequency
3–5 sets	5–15 repetitions or as duration/time.	Variable depending on the outcome goals: Explosive, controlled, or focus on eccentric loading or concentric loading. For example: 2-0-2 4-1-2 2-1-4 2-4-2 1-1-2 Or prescribed duration	Progressive from body weight to loaded. Must lead to an overload/repetition maximum on the exercises. Consider the force–velocity curve for optimal loading in relation to targets. Progression with dumbbells, barbells, medicine balls and cables, for example. Always performed with quality. Brace and move.	3–4 x each week 2–4 specific core exercises selected within whole-body strength programme, which also addresses the core and posterior chain. More likely to involve whole-body compound movement patterns. Separate core sessions may also be completed in addition to functional whole-body strength work.

143

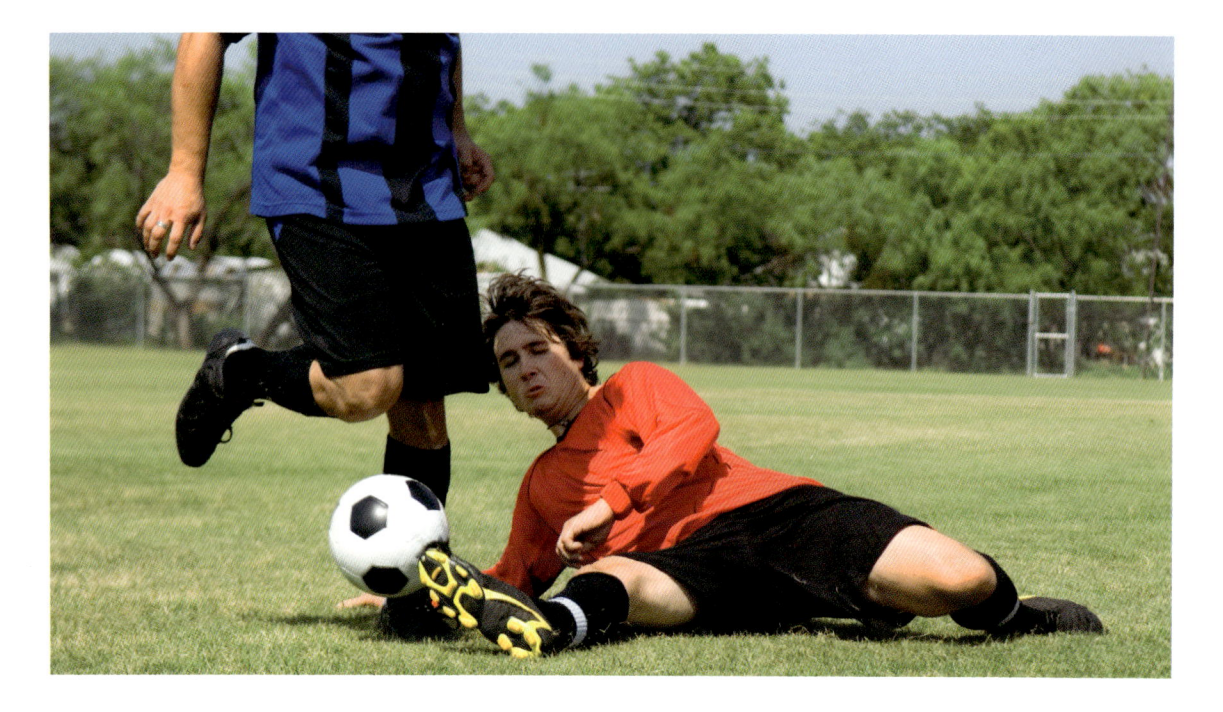

APPLIED CORE CONDITIONING: PROGRAMMING, PRESCRIPTION

A tackle in football is a complex movement, requiring a good range of movement plus spinal control, co-contraction of the lower limbs, in addition to accuracy, strength and agility. If contact occurs, the body must be able to react and be robust as the force goes through the body. A weakness in the core, sling systems or posterior chain may lead to muscular injury.

swing then superset with a volleyball spike drill; or the resisted cable shuffle then release to complete some defensive slides or 1v1 game in basketball. Supersetting these athletic movements with core activation will mimic the demands placed upon the individual during training and games, which will help them become robust and strong and also adds variation, fun and a good stimulus to training.

Seated Events

Horse riding, motor racing, motorbike speedway, motocross, cycling, BMX, bobsleigh, rowing, kayak, canoeing.

I have had the pleasure of working with a British GT3 motor-racing driver for a number of years now. He was getting delayed-onset headaches after competing because of the G-force created at high speeds in the car. Although he was fine during the race, he would often experience an almost a whiplash-like effect 24 to 48 hours later. It was something he wanted to address and prevent if possible. Specific neck-strengthening work seemed to alleviate the problem, while specific seated strengthening work improved his core strength, and functional isometric strength in a seated position during his driving also strengthened his kinetic chain. He is exposed to high torque forces on the track and his ability to cope with this and to regulate his foot and lower limb control while in a seated position, to bleed on and off the accelerator effectively at corners (monitored via the team's data analysis technology), has also improved due to some stretch-shortening cycle conditioning/activation work, alongside his specific core and lower-limb strength work. Such improvements can gain a few 100ths of a second, which over a 2-hour race can be the difference between winning and losing. Because of his driving position during a race, many of the exercises were completed in seated. The skill in S&C is to ensure that there is a transfer from the gym into actual performance. Not only did the neck-strengthening work help, but thoracic spine mobility work, seated BOSU medicine ball work and Paloff press cable work also helped to strengthen his kinetic chain. If one of these stimuli had been omitted, maybe the post-race headaches would still have gone away, but, as a result of a fully comprehensive programme and a whole-body approach, the driver is now a highly conditioned individual.

Horse riding, motorbike speedway, motocross, BMX, bobsleigh, kayaking, canoeing and cycling also place significant demands on the core and posterior chain. Body load is high when a cyclist rider rises out of the saddle during a hill climb, or a horse rider does the same when galloping, or when a BMX or motocross rider is managing the bumps of challenging terrain while retaining control of their bike, leaning in as they accelerate. Their feet and hands may be the only points of contact on the bike, and they have to control where it moves, how fast it goes and any tricks along the way. The core is activated when limbs move, so, in this hip-flexed seated position, it is important to ensure that the athlete has a good strength foundation. Being in a long-term flexed position can shorten the muscles, so it may be that exercise selection and programming for the seated athlete would look at hip extension mobility work or loading through a Bulgarian squat, for example, to ensure that mobility is maintained and protected. If hip flexors become tight, this can transfer to a pelvic tilt, low back pain and a change in biomechanics, which may lead to over-use issues or injury.

Of course, the horse, the terrain and other drivers or riders make these sports unpredictable, so having a reactive strength capacity is important. For cyclists, alternate leg work that is functional is important, along with a strong kinetic chain, power and strength in the legs, excellent stability in the hips, glutes and core, and of course a strong yet mobile lumbar spine, to cope with hours in a flexed position on the bike. It is clear from observing a cyclist that the core does not work in isolation; instead, it must work as part of the global unit, stabilizing the spine and lumbo-pelvic hip region and helping to create force as the legs power on and the arms and upper body stabilize on the handlebars.

In a kayak or canoe, when a paddle is used to control and steer, the athlete must be able to stabilize through their spine, whilst in an upright or flexed position. They may even move into extension as they resist the water to turn in a rapid, and this requires excellent isometric and rotational strength, as well as excellent upper-body strength and endurance capacity. The resistance of the rapids adds a reactive strength requirement, which needs to be considered when training.

Rowers tend to be high-performance, self-driven athletes and low back pain is common in this group. A very good core-strengthening programme is essential as an injury prevention strategy, in addition to a compound strength programme with more performance-based lifts based around strength and power. In 2016, *World Rowing* published an article by Dr Fiona Wilson, addressing back pain in rowers. This is a very valuable resource, specifically for rowers, and Dr Wilson's philosophy mirrors the concepts presented in this book:

> *Some key points in low back pain rehabilitation and prevention programmes are that the body should be considered as a 'whole system' and that all joints interact together. Small changes and compensation in some systems (such as stiff hips or poor back muscle endurance) have an influence on the whole athlete. Another area, which is often poorly addressed, is 'specificity' in rehabilitation, especially the 'core'. An approach which does not consider the movement patterns required in rowing with an over-emphasis on static strengthening is of limited use. Dynamic activities,*

APPLIED CORE CONDITIONING: PROGRAMMING, PRESCRIPTION

which encourage the lower back to move normally in rowing patterns, are the most appropriate.

Thoracic mobility, as well as a healthy, strong and mobile lumbar spine, is important in these seated events. The glutes also play a significant role in stabilizing, so they need to be well conditioned. Hamstrings may become tight as well as hip flexors, so the good morning exercise, Romanian dead lift and Bulgarian squats may be used in exercise selection, to complement the core conditioning and to ensure a good range of movement through the hamstrings in the posterior chain and the hip flexors anteriorly. Once again, progress is made towards whole-body movement patterns that condition other parts of the body, but always ensuring that strength and mobility are maintained through the core, and that the exercises are specific to the movement patterns required for the sport.

Using external aids, such as cables and bands, as well as medicine balls and suspension training, is also relevant. One major consideration with programming and exercise selection is for the core to be braced and static but for the limbs to be moving, which mimics what often happens for this group of athletes. Whether it is the arms turning the wheel in the racing car, or holding the reins of the horse, or a paddle or oar, the core and trunk must be strong and stable.

Seated events demand good stability but also require control of the extremities, whether steering a wheel, handlebar or paddle, or cycling with the legs. The isometric capacity and strength of the core are essential to ensure that the athlete reduces the incidence of low back pain. This balance – between

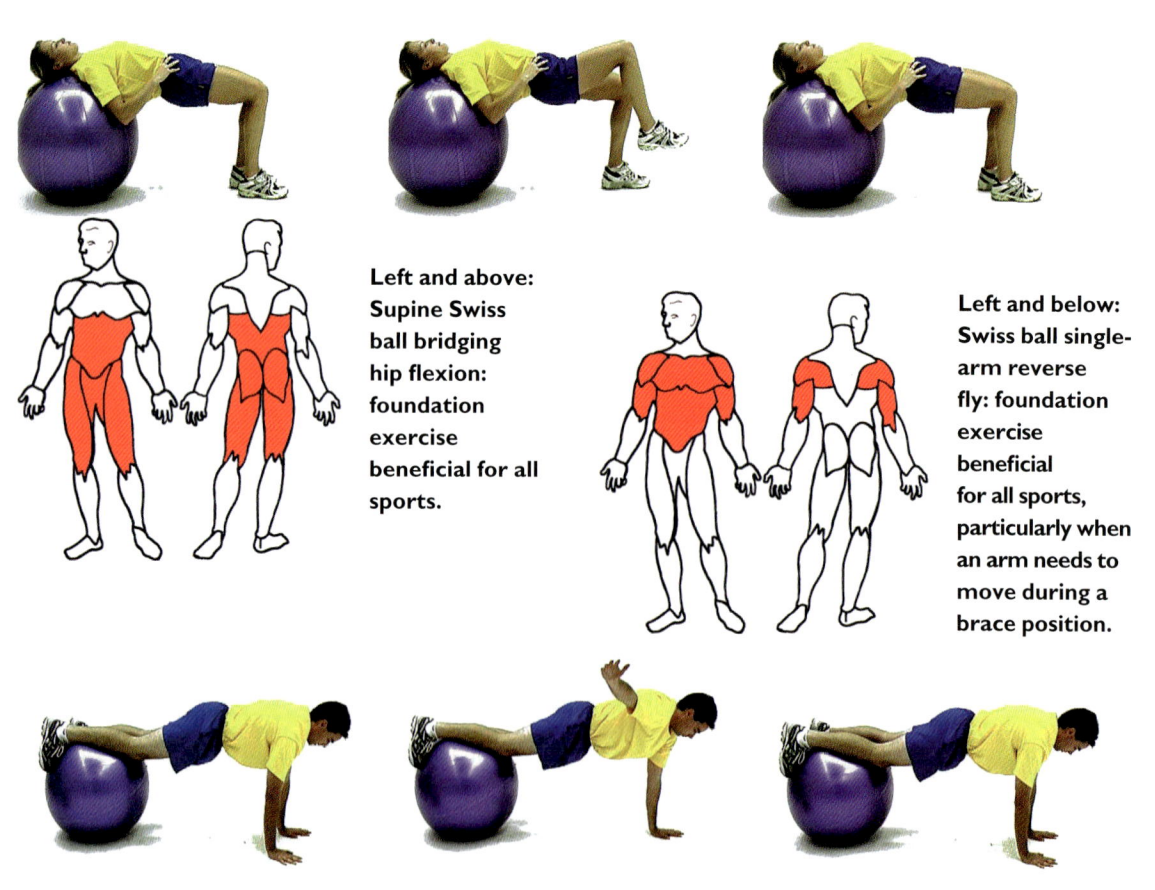

Left and above: Supine Swiss ball bridging hip flexion: foundation exercise beneficial for all sports.

Left and below: Swiss ball single-arm reverse fly: foundation exercise beneficial for all sports, particularly when an arm needs to move during a brace position.

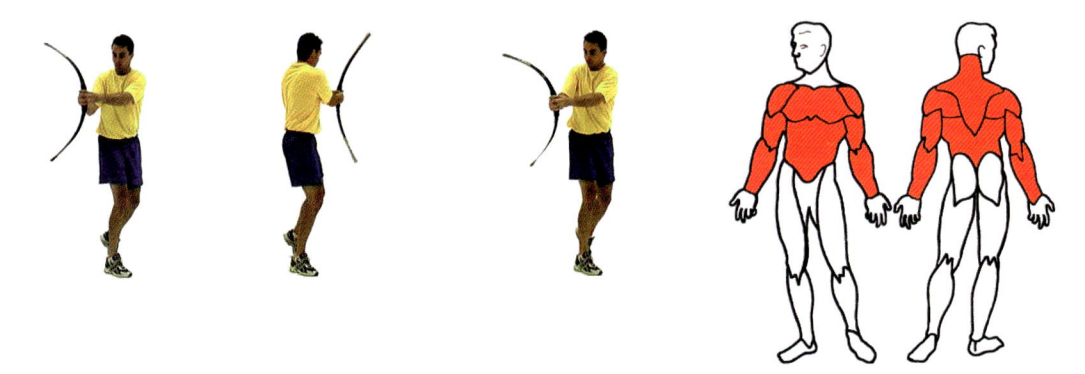

APPLIED CORE CONDITIONING: PROGRAMMING, PRESCRIPTION

Body blade rotation: foundation exercise beneficial for all sports, particularly when the arms need to move during a brace position and the core experiences reactive demands (horse riding, **BMX**, motor racing, kayak, motorbike speedway and motocross).

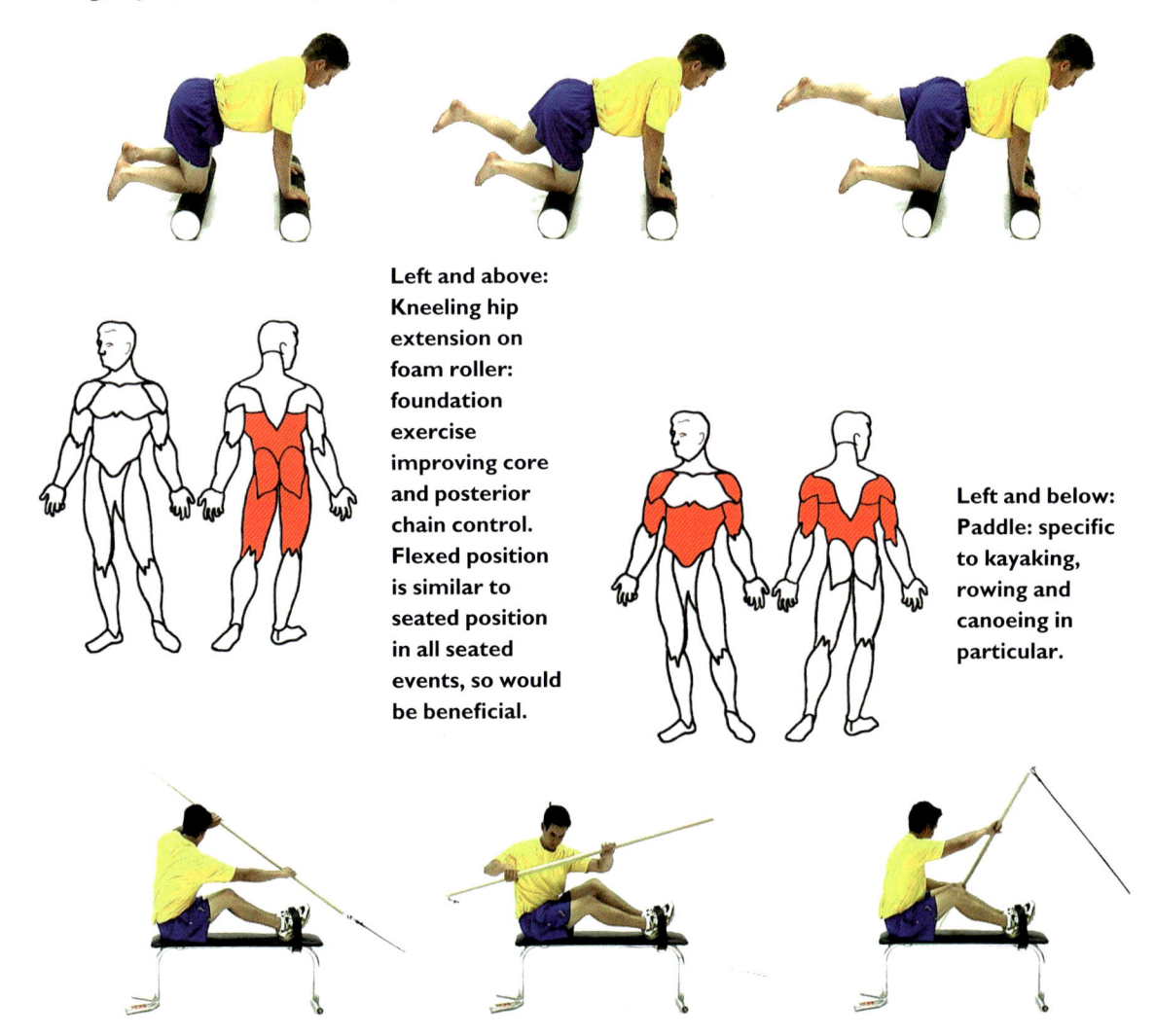

Left and above: Kneeling hip extension on foam roller: foundation exercise improving core and posterior chain control. Flexed position is similar to seated position in all seated events, so would be beneficial.

Left and below: Paddle: specific to kayaking, rowing and canoeing in particular.

147

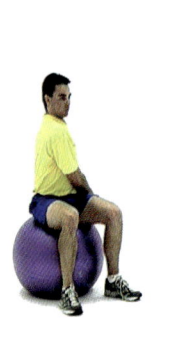

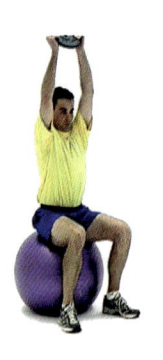

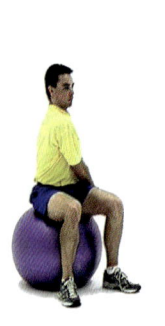

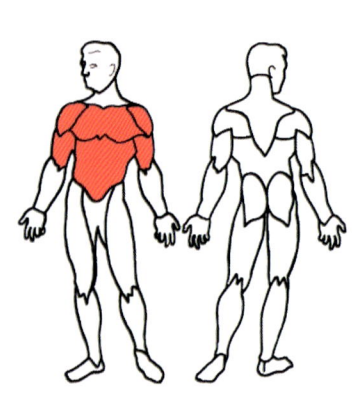

APPLIED CORE CONDITIONING: PROGRAMMING, PRESCRIPTION

Seated wood chop: all seated events but particularly water sports (canoe, kayaking and rowing).

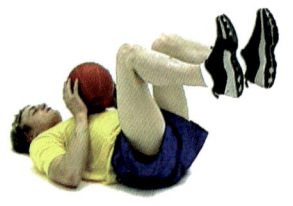

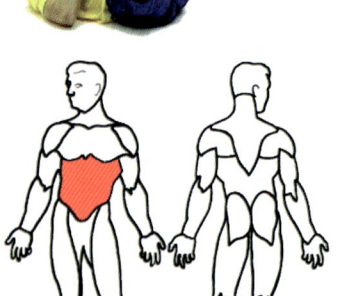

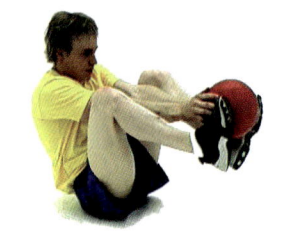

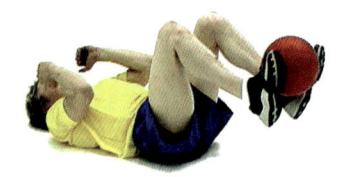

Medicine ball sit-up hip flexion: seated position as flexed, appropriate for all seated events and places concentric and eccentric load through the core.

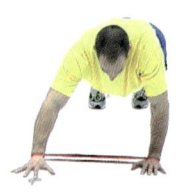

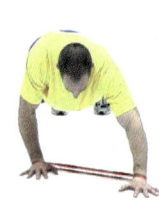

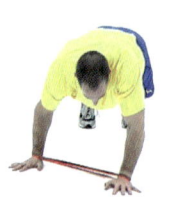

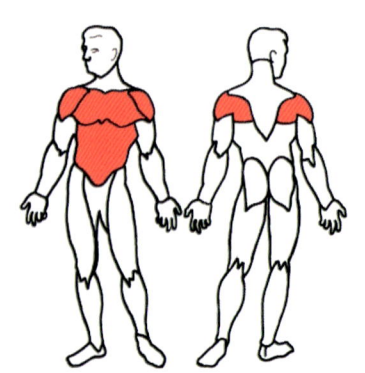

Band prone walk circuit: cycling, BMX, motocross and motorbike speedway.

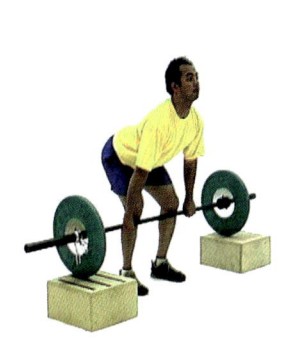

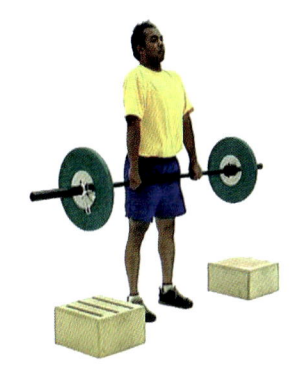

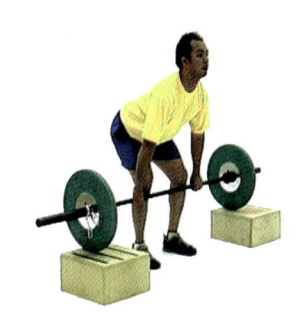

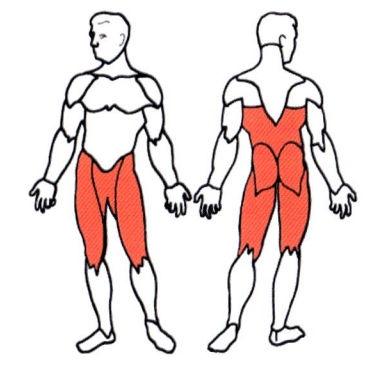

APPLIED CORE CONDITIONING: PROGRAMMING, PRESCRIPTION

Dead lift (from hang): excellent posterior chain exercise, beneficial for horse riding, motor racing, motorbike speedway, motocross, cycling, **BMX**, bobsleigh, rowing, kayaking, canoeing.

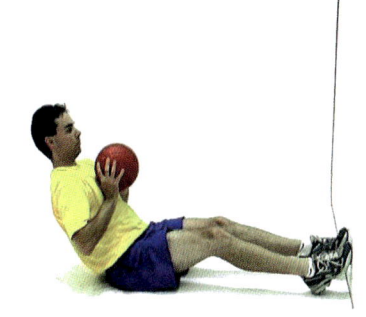

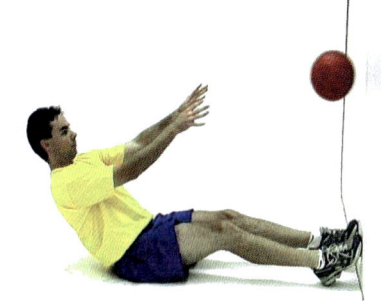

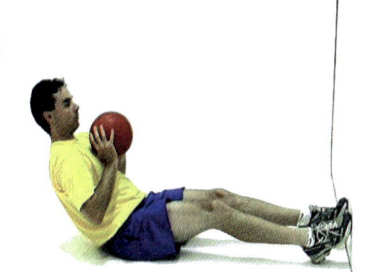

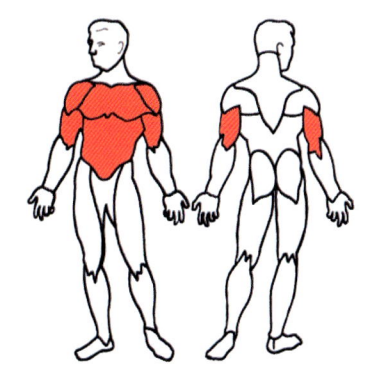

Medicine ball throw, with arms moving and isometric hold: horse riding, motor racing, motorbike speedway, motocross, cycling, **BMX**, bobsleigh, rowing, kayaking, canoeing.

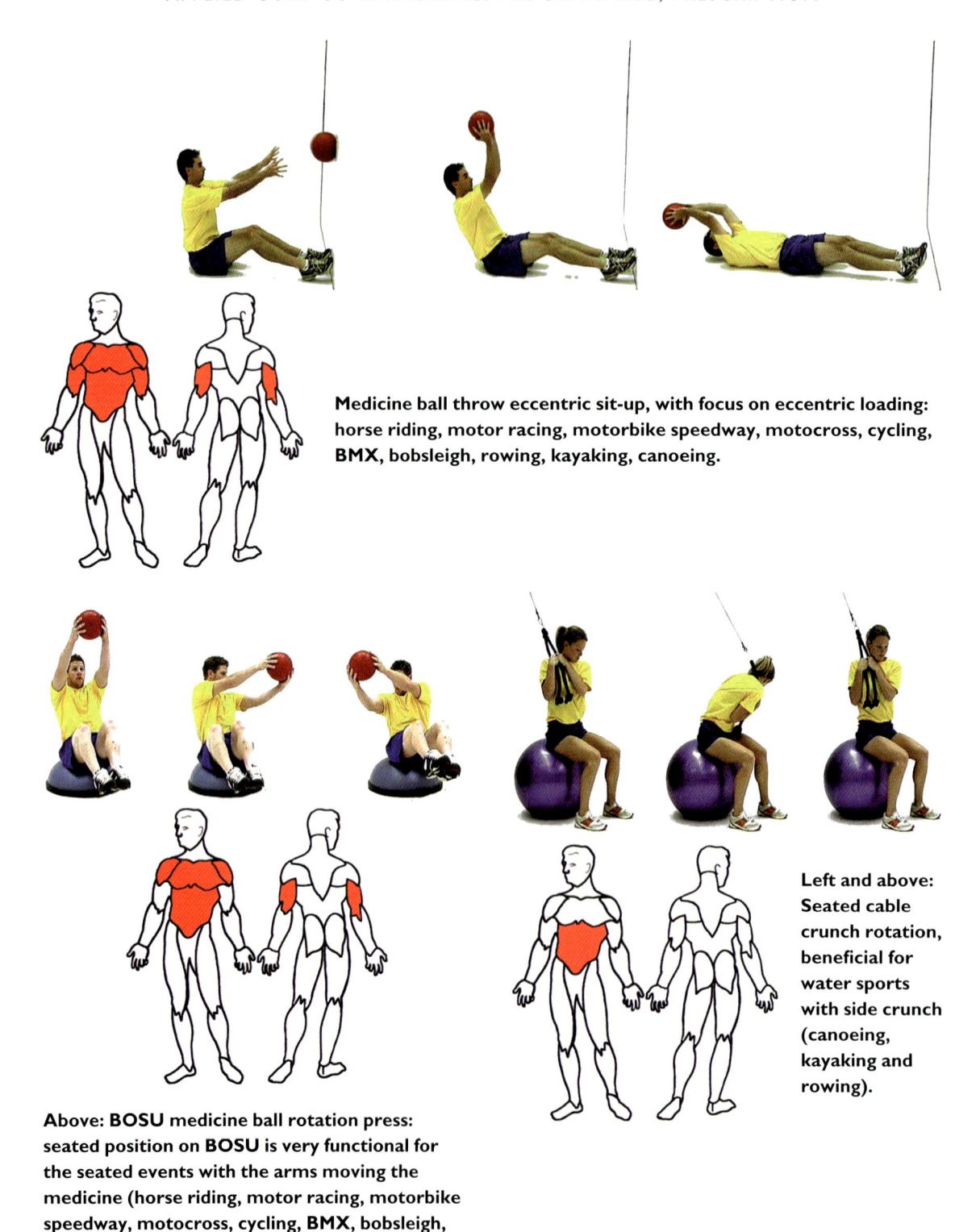

APPLIED CORE CONDITIONING: PROGRAMMING, PRESCRIPTION

Medicine ball throw eccentric sit-up, with focus on eccentric loading: horse riding, motor racing, motorbike speedway, motocross, cycling, **BMX**, bobsleigh, rowing, kayaking, canoeing.

Above: **BOSU** medicine ball rotation press: seated position on **BOSU** is very functional for the seated events with the arms moving the medicine (horse riding, motor racing, motorbike speedway, motocross, cycling, **BMX**, bobsleigh, rowing, kayaking, canoeing).

Left and above: Seated cable crunch rotation, beneficial for water sports with side crunch (canoeing, kayaking and rowing).

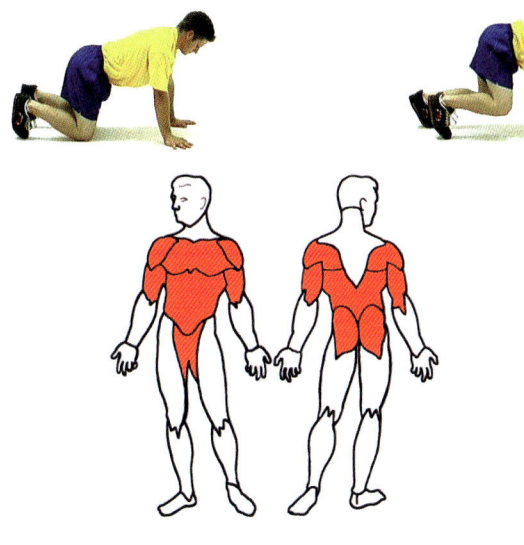

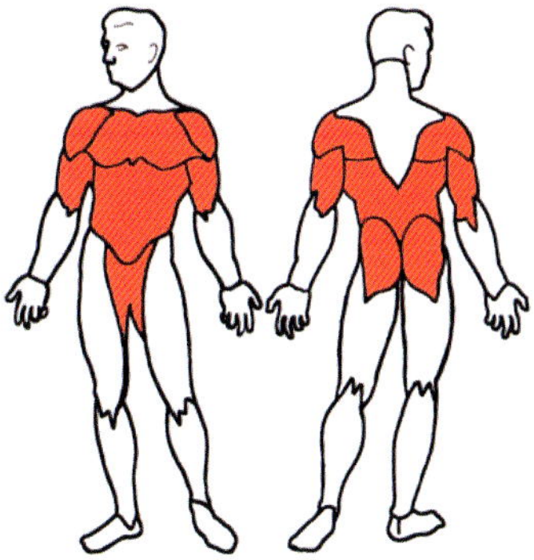

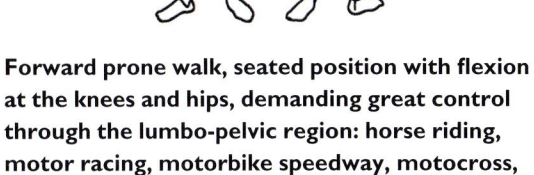

APPLIED CORE CONDITIONING: PROGRAMMING, PRESCRIPTION

Forward prone walk, seated position with flexion at the knees and hips, demanding great control through the lumbo-pelvic region: horse riding, motor racing, motorbike speedway, motocross, cycling, **BMX**, bobsleigh, rowing, kayaking, canoeing.

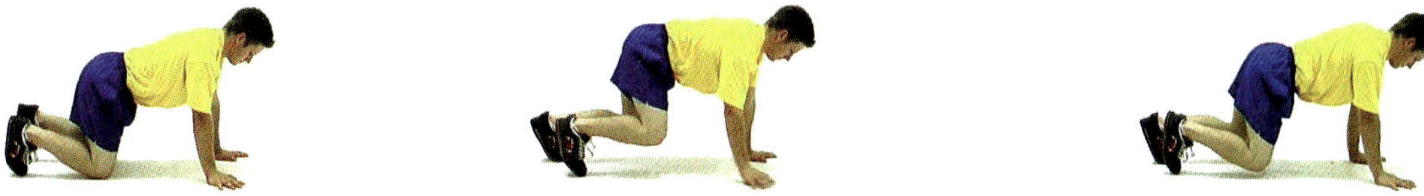

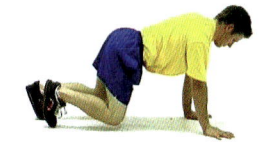

Backward prone walk, seated position with flexion at the knees and hips, demanding great control through the lumbo-pelvic region: horse riding, motor racing, motorbike speedway, motocross, cycling, **BMX**, bobsleigh, rowing, kayaking, canoeing.

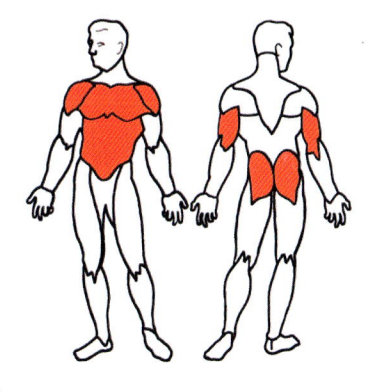

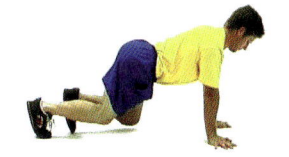

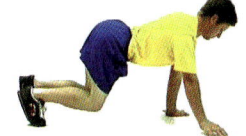

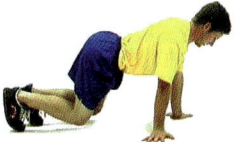

maintaining a strong core and posterior chain and ensuring mobility – is important. Being in a flexed position on a bicycle for hours on end and creating the necessary power output in the legs requires excellent conditioning. If the lower back and core are not strong enough, then shearing may occur, or increased spinal loading may cause problems and pain. The neural system is being stretched and challenged and so a neural mobility and lumbar spine/thoracic spine mobility plan should be prescribed for overall health and wellbeing. These athletes are upright or in a dynamic flexed/extended position for training and competition and need to be strong to cope, but they also should have in place a mobility plan, spinal mobility, flexion, extension and rotation work, as well and perhaps overhead squats for thoracic mobility. Foam rolling for myofascial release would also be useful to help release the muscles and aid recovery.

Exercise selection: the seated event exercises vary from seated or standing isometric holds to the limbs, arms or legs moving. Many of the exercises have the athlete in a triple flexed position with hips, knees and ankles flexed, as in the forward and backward prone walk, for example. If the athlete were flipped by 90 degrees in this case, they would

151

Programme design and prescription for core conditioning for seated events

Sets	Repetitions	Tempo	Load	Frequency
3–5 sets	5–30 repetitions or time/duration. Depends on nature of the sport: power-based/explosive or endurance-based.	Variable depending on the outcome goals: focus more on stability and isometric work then progress to dynamic/explosive work with extremities loaded or moving: 2-0-2 4-1-2 2-1-4 2-4-2 1-1-2 Or prescribed duration: 30 seconds for example.	Progressive but must lead to an overload/repetition maximum on the exercises through reps or fatigue from duration. Consider the force–velocity curve for optimal loading in relation to targets. Always performed with quality.	3–4 x each week 4–6 exercises selected depending on phase of training and other demands. Whole-body conditioning to complement core conditioning is necessary for overall conditioning/performance and injury prevention.

be in their seated position on their bike or horse, or in their canoe. This makes these positions quite functional for these sports. The legs or arms can be dynamic, moving and mimicking the movements required in the sport and the core and pelvis may be fixed. In addition, compound exercises can be used, such the dead lift, in which power and strength are required through the posterior chain and lower limbs.

Endurance and Linear Events

Running, triathlon, athletics, Nordic skiing, hiking, rowing, archery, skiing, fencing, gymnastics, sailing, speed skating, swimming, hurdles.

It is clear that running economy can be improved with an increase in core strength, and of course the load demands in running, hiking, triathlon and Nordic skiing are similar in nature, with lower-body movement and arm swings. The job of the core musculature and lumbo-pelvic region is to stabilize the spine as the athlete moves. If there is an imbalance or weakness, there may be shearing and movement around the spine, which can lead to injury and pain. The athlete needs to be strong enough to deal with the constant repetitive loading that these endurance events require. Such events, in which the tonic nature of the core is called upon to stabilize while the body propels itself along, present a risk of over-use injury. A strong kinetic chain will help reduce injury and ensure a good resilience.

Nordic skiing demands immensely strong legs, as well as a powerful upper body to push along and carve through the snow. Some of the highest-ever VO_2 max results have been recorded on Nordic skiers (and cyclists) – at 80–90ml/kg/min – demonstrating an exceptional aerobic capacity, but these athletes also need to be strong and robust to reduce the incidence of injury and to aid performance.

In fencing, a competitor may lunge forward to score a point or recoil to avoid being hit; both movements demand good core strength and reactive capacity. Similarly, when a hurdler sprints and explodes to get over the hurdles in sequence, the trunk and core are required to stabilize the spine, so, the stronger the lumbo-pelvic region, the more efficient the athlete can be. They need a good

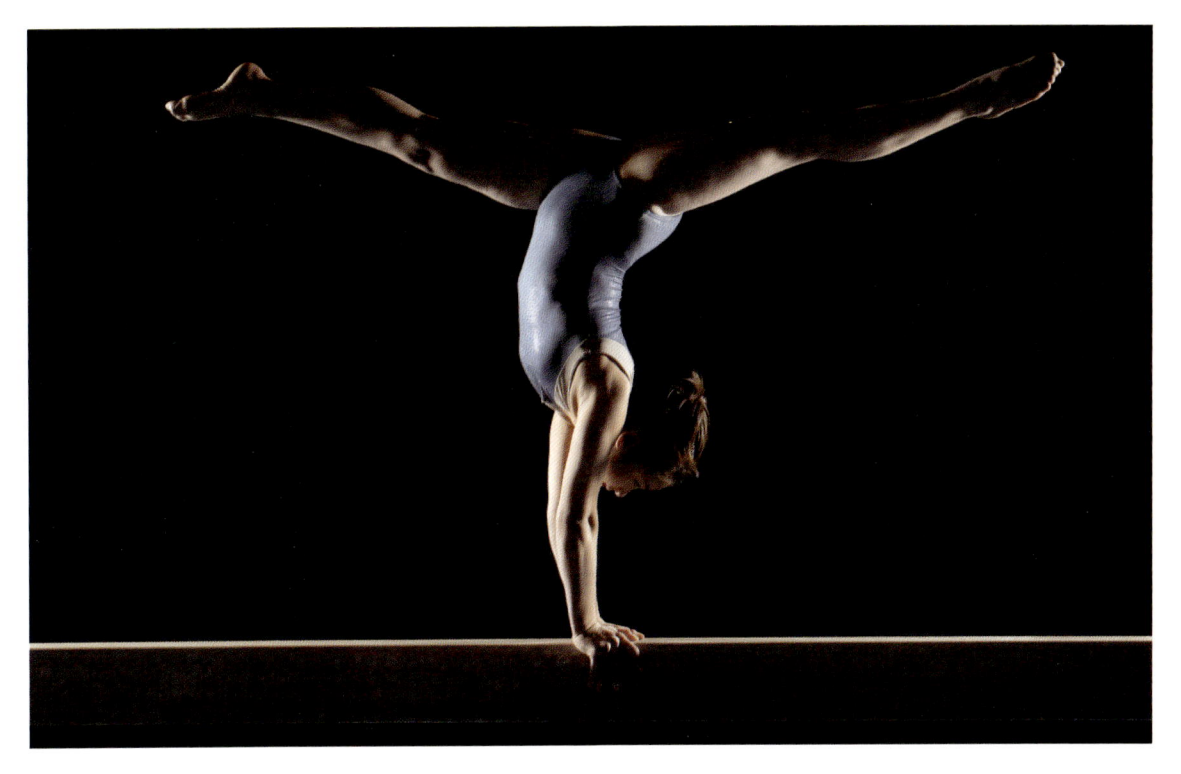

APPLIED CORE CONDITIONING: PROGRAMMING, PRESCRIPTION

A gymnast demonstrating great whole-body strength. The core and lumbo-pelvic hip region must be strong, yet they must also have excellent mobility and flexibility.

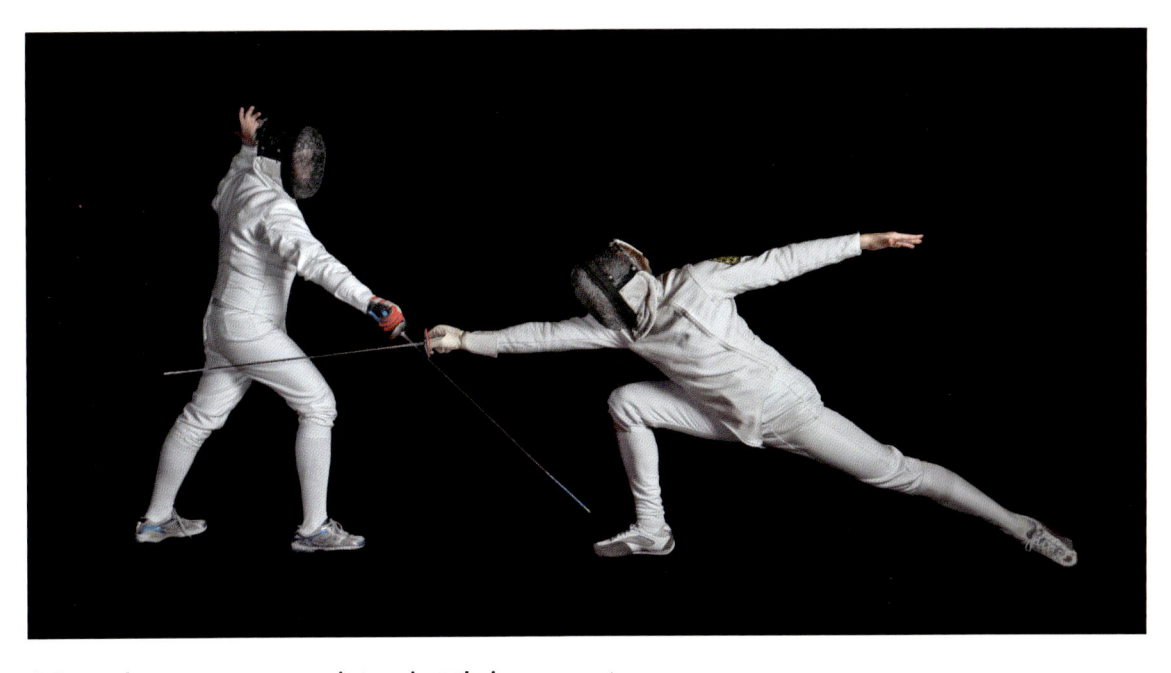

A fencer lunges to score a point against their opponent.

APPLIED CORE CONDITIONING: PROGRAMMING, PRESCRIPTION

stretch-shortening cycle for power and explosiveness, in addition to a strong core and mobility for the hip drive over the hurdle. The common theme is that a balance between strength and mobility leads to a more resilient and robust athlete. The practitioner must select the most sports-specific appropriate exercises to challenge the individual once the foundation strength and activation have been achieved.

The tonic nature of the core is important with endurance events, but, if there in insufficient capacity in the lower limbs, the body will break down eventually in the weakest part of the chain. Once again, the core-strengthening exercises must be complemented by additional lower limb strengthening and compound exercises, to allow for a coordinated effort in endurance or linear events. As in the conditioning exercises for the seated

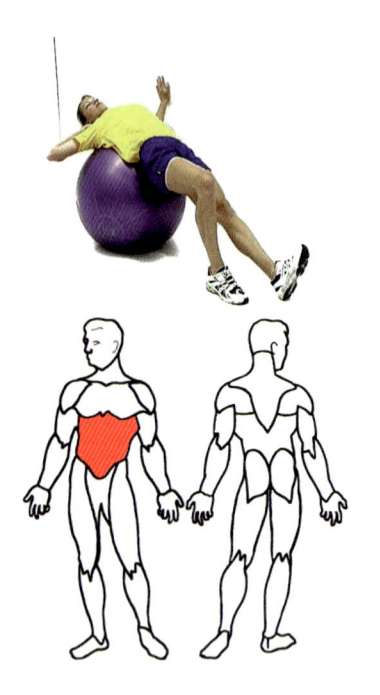

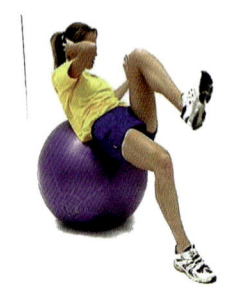

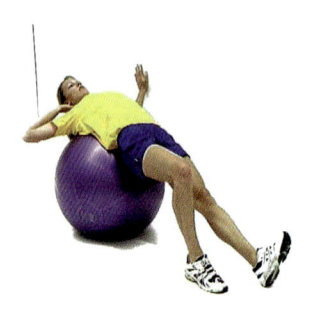

Swiss ball sit-up rotation: the sling system movement is good for hurdlers, Nordic skiers, speed skating and swimming.

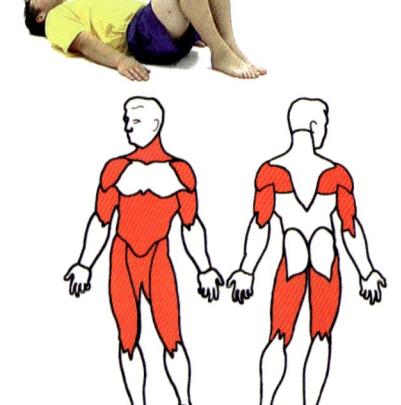

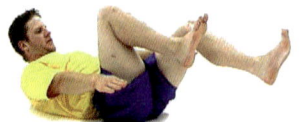

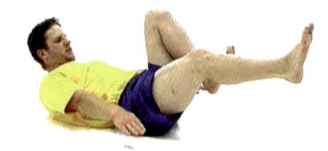

Alternating hip flexion extension: alternating leg movement is very functional for linear and endurance events (running, triathlon, athletics, Nordic skiing, hiking, rowing, archery, skiing, fencing, gymnastics, sailing, speed skating, swimming, hurdles).

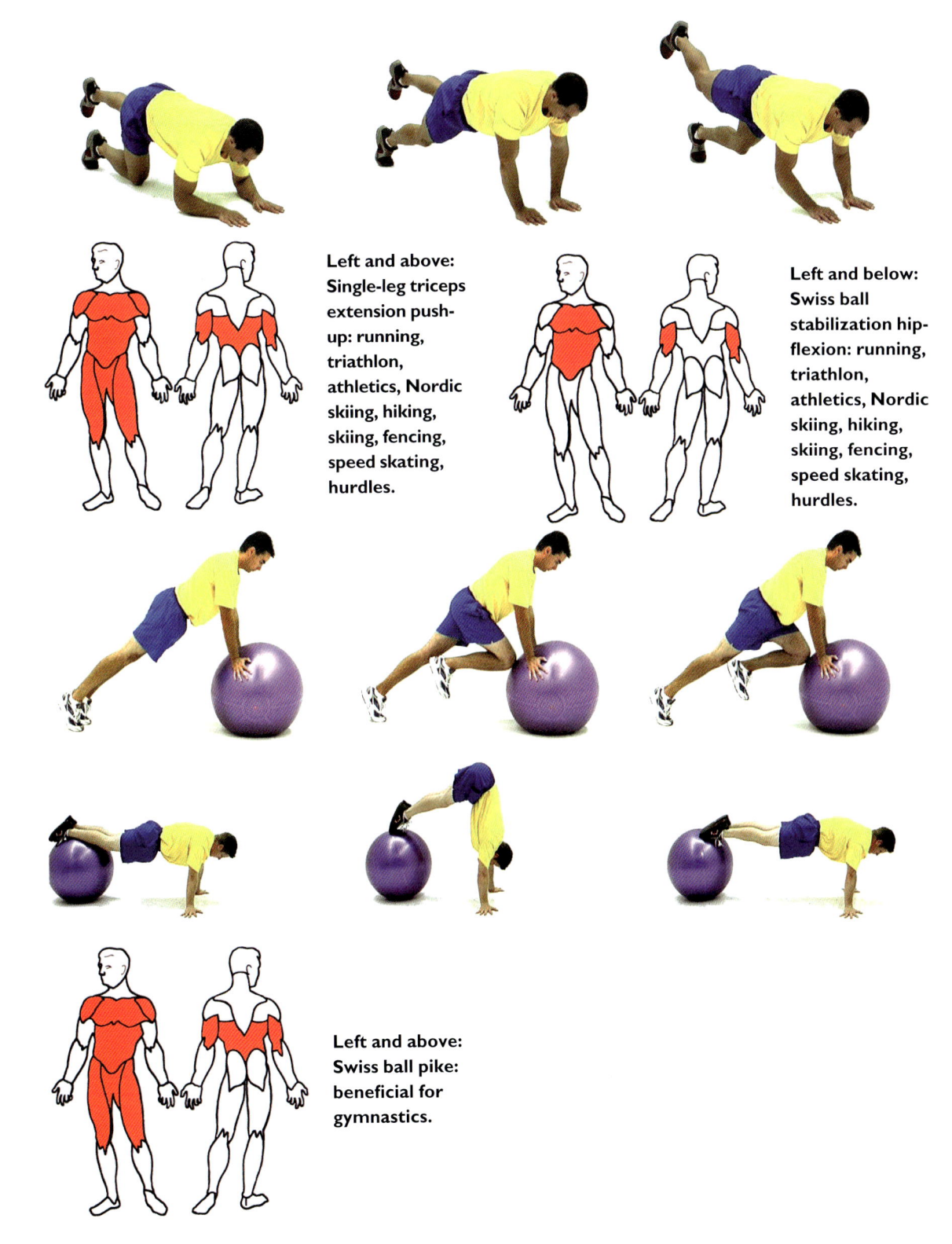

APPLIED CORE CONDITIONING: PROGRAMMING, PRESCRIPTION

Left and above: Single-leg triceps extension push-up: running, triathlon, athletics, Nordic skiing, hiking, skiing, fencing, speed skating, hurdles.

Left and below: Swiss ball stabilization hip-flexion: running, triathlon, athletics, Nordic skiing, hiking, skiing, fencing, speed skating, hurdles.

Left and above: Swiss ball pike: beneficial for gymnastics.

155

APPLIED CORE CONDITIONING: PROGRAMMING, PRESCRIPTION

Left and above: Single-leg bridging on a bench: running, triathlon, athletics, Nordic skiing, hiking, rowing, archery, skiing, fencing, gymnastics, sailing, speed skating.

Left and above: Hip flexion rotation: running, triathlon, athletics, Nordic skiing, hiking, fencing, speed skating.

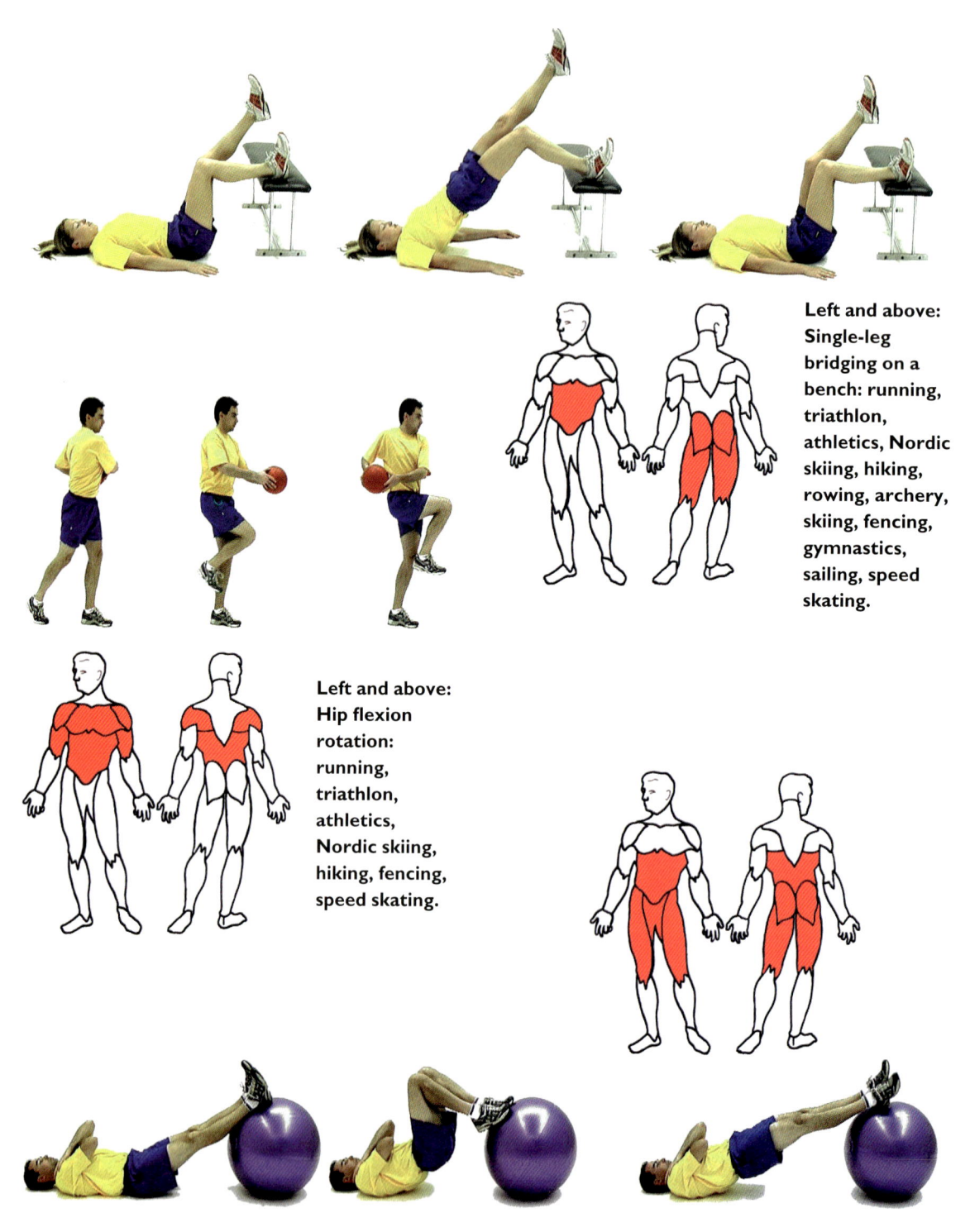

Swiss ball curls: running, triathlon, athletics, Nordic skiing, hiking, rowing, archery, skiing, fencing, gymnastics, sailing, speed skating, swimming, hurdles.

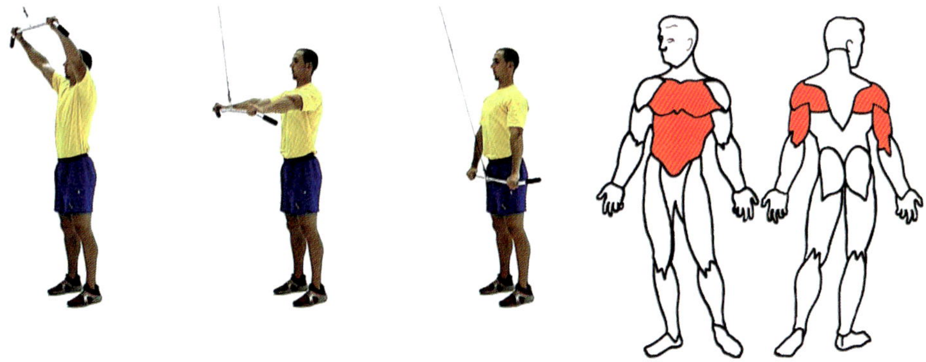

APPLIED CORE CONDITIONING: PROGRAMMING, PRESCRIPTION

Cable straight-arm lateral pulldown: sailing, swimming, Nordic skiing and skiing.

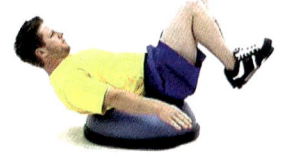

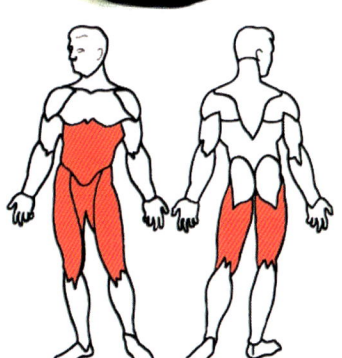

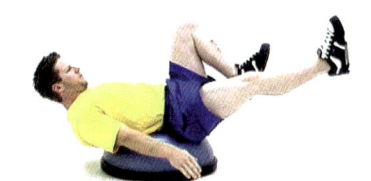

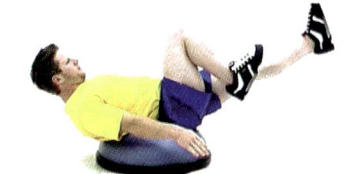

BOSU alternating hip flexion-extension: running, triathlon, athletics, Nordic skiing, hiking, skiing, hurdles.

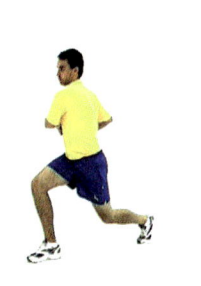

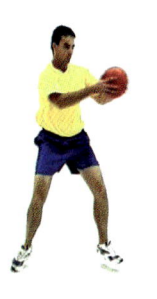

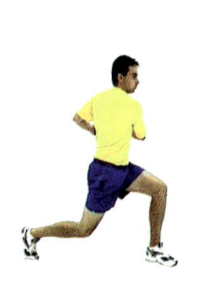

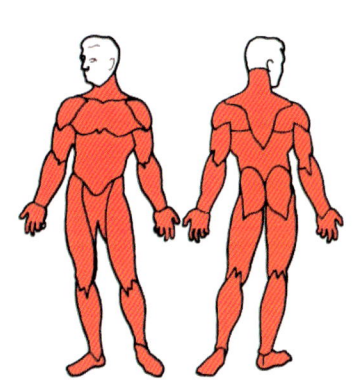

Split jumps rotation: fencing, Nordic skiing, speed skating.

APPLIED CORE CONDITIONING: PROGRAMMING, PRESCRIPTION

Above: High pull: running, triathlon, athletics, Nordic skiing, hiking, rowing, archery, skiing, fencing, gymnastics, sailing, speed skating, swimming, hurdles.

Left and above: Lunge walk rotation: running, triathlon, athletics, Nordic skiing, hiking, skiing, fencing, gymnastics, speed skating, swimming, hurdles.

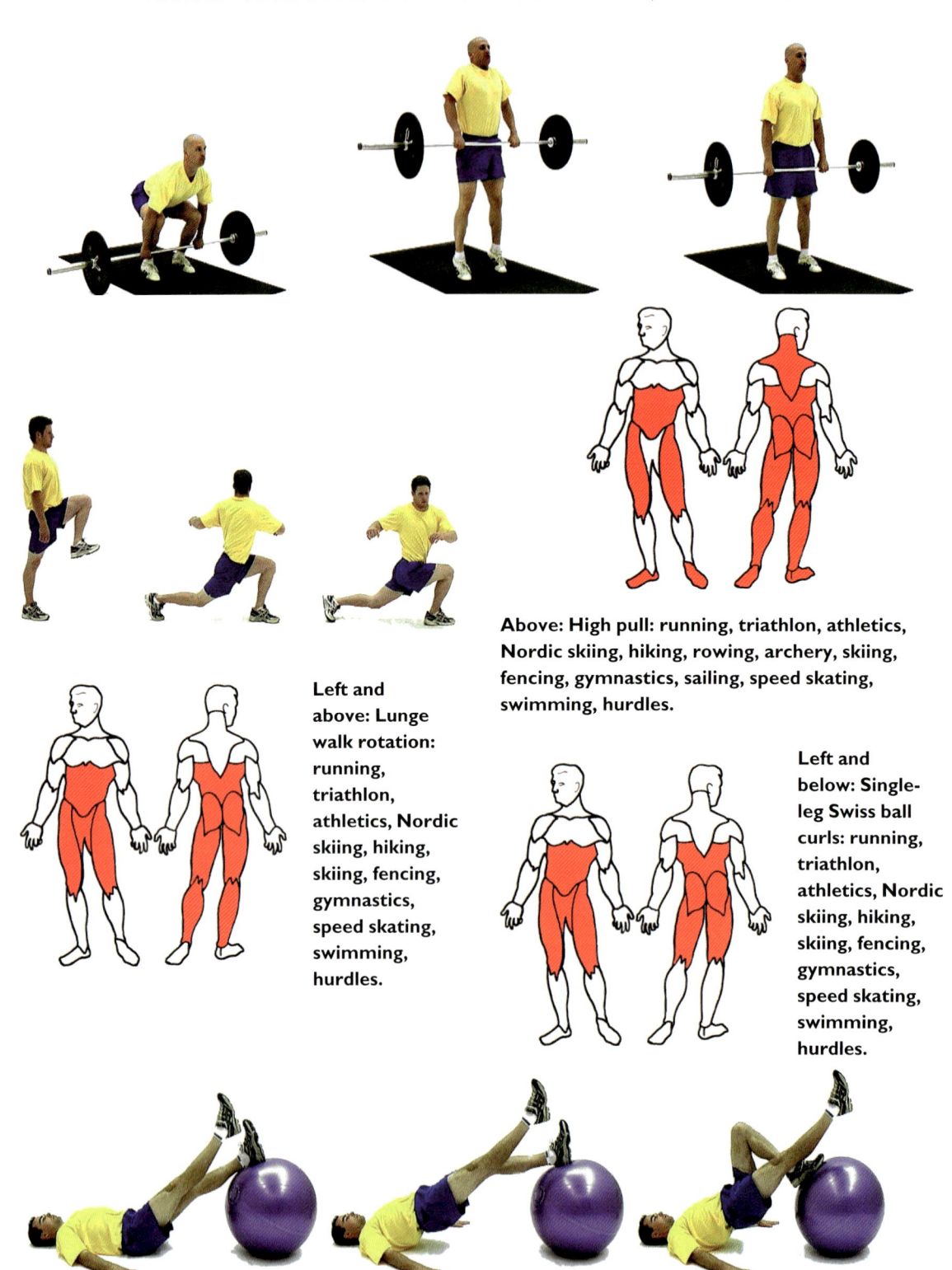

Left and below: Single-leg Swiss ball curls: running, triathlon, athletics, Nordic skiing, hiking, skiing, fencing, gymnastics, speed skating, swimming, hurdles.

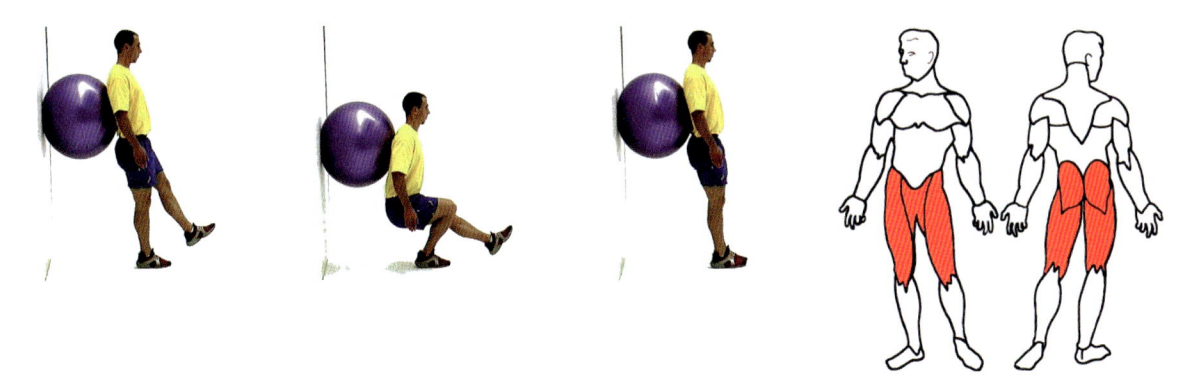

APPLIED CORE CONDITIONING: PROGRAMMING, PRESCRIPTION

Stability ball single-leg squat: running, triathlon, athletics, Nordic skiing, hiking, skiing, fencing, gymnastics, speed skating, swimming, hurdles.

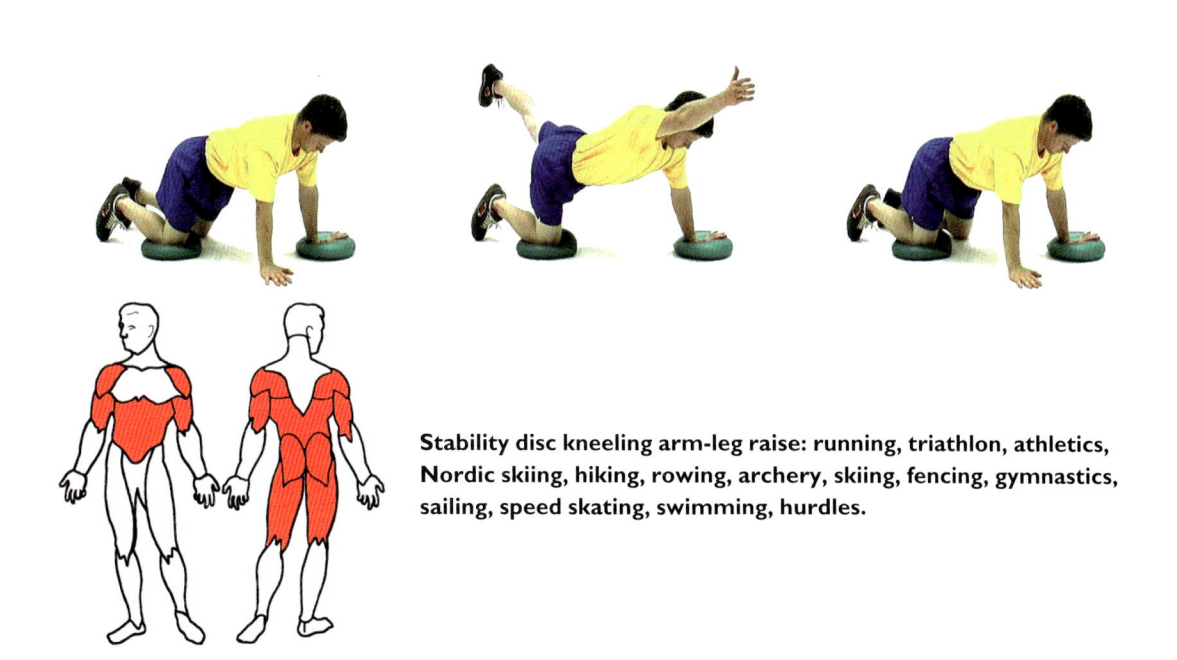

Stability disc kneeling arm-leg raise: running, triathlon, athletics, Nordic skiing, hiking, rowing, archery, skiing, fencing, gymnastics, sailing, speed skating, swimming, hurdles.

events, the core will often be static in an isometric hold, and the limbs will be moving. It is important to consider this when prescribing and programming appropriate exercises.

The exercise selection for endurance and linear events is based more around isometric control through the lumbo-pelvic region, but it often involves a limb moving and the sling systems at work, often with alternating arms/legs, in addition to some lunge patterns and certainly some lower-limb posterior chain work. The aim is to ensure not only a sound core foundation and capacity, but also conditioning for the associated musculature for the loading pattern required, in other words, alternate leg or arm lunge patterns. These exercise programmes would benefit from additional compound strength work for the lower limbs or upper limbs, depending on the sport. More isometric strength through the core can be developed by standing in a braced position and completing some single-leg flexion and

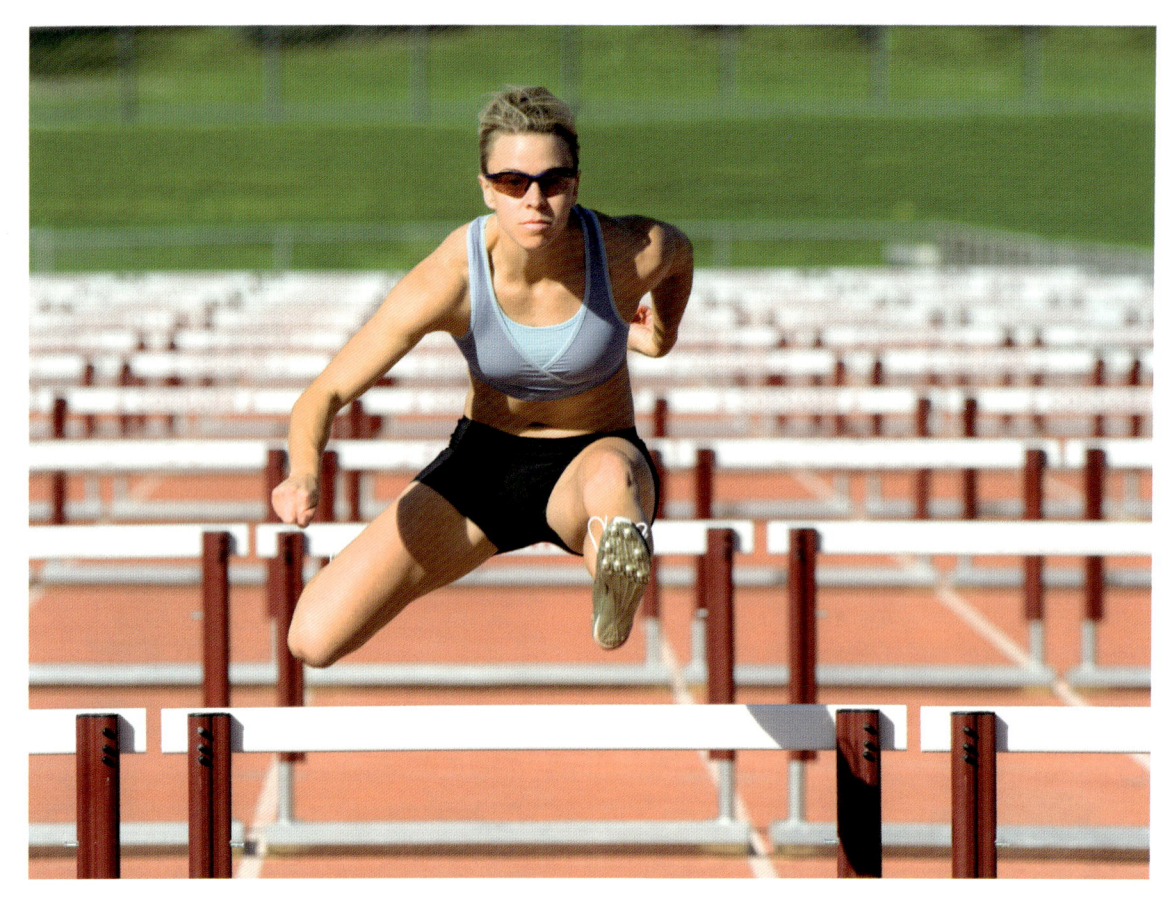

A hurdler demands excellent stability through the spine and core, despite her lower limbs accelerating and flexing and extending as they jump over the hurdles. Excellent coordination is required as well as strength through the sling systems and an excellent stretch-shortening cycle capacity.

extension, alternate cable rows, or lunge patterns, with resistance from a band or cable machine. These exercises will also develop strength, stability and power in the limbs. Once again, the importance of compound movements in sport and the resultant applied strength development must not be underestimated.

Exercise selection: once again, isometric holds are included but with an arm or leg moving. Often, it is good practice to alternate legs or arm movements, to mimic the movement patterns and demands of the sport. Resistance can be added via bands or cables, kettle bells, dumbbells or medicine balls, and instability can be increased via a BOSU, suspension training, balance cushion or Swiss ball. There are also a number of general conditioning exercises that are the 'gold standard' for running-based events. These include Swiss ball curls, alternating hip flexion-extension and stability disc kneeling arm-leg raise. These can all work from a basic foundation level and be progressed as the athlete develops control and strength through the core. Compound movements that are more demanding and metabolic can also be included, for example, the high pull and split jumps rotation.

Programme design and prescription for core conditioning for endurance and linear events

Sets	Repetitions	Tempo	Load	Frequency
3–5 sets	5–12 repetitions or time/duration. Depends on the nature of the sport: power-based/explosive or endurance-based. Some sports may need both.	Variable depending on the outcome goals: focus more on stability and isometric work with extremities loaded or moving: 2-0-2 4-1-2 2-1-4 2-4-2 1-1-2 Or prescribed duration	Progressive but must lead to an overload/repetition maximum on the exercises through reps or fatigue from duration. Consider the force–velocity curve for optimal loading in relation to targets. Always performed with quality.	3–4 x each week 3–4 exercises selected depending on phase of training and other demands. Whole-body conditioning to complement the core conditioning and mirror the demands of the sport when possible.

Programme Design Summary

No matter what the sport or activity, a foundation of core strength needs to be developed and established before more complex movements are introduced. There are no short cuts to this. If the demands placed upon the body are too high and the appropriate strength has not yet been established, loading will occur through the spine, which is clearly undesirable. However, once the foundation is strong enough, the applied conditioning of the core can be progressed, to include very sport-specific activities.

Mimicking the movement pattern, and becoming stronger and more efficient with that movement, should improve performance and also help reduce the incidence of injury and damage through overuse. This is especially the case in events that require repeated movement patterns, such as rowing, tennis, kayaking and canoe. The link between the body through the core is also highlighted in this respect, particularly in the seated events, where the legs may be doing much of the work, while the lumbo-pelvic region and core are stabilizing and creating power. This link allows the body to work efficiently at the highest level. The athlete must ensure that there is no leakage of strength or power from the body and that every ounce of energy and efficiency is utilized for performance. It is also important to recognize that, in many of these examples, there is a crossover to all sports (although some may be more specific to one sport than to another). Completing challenging and appropriate core-strengthening exercises, in addition to compound exercises, will help establish a strong core.

In my basketball-playing days, I remember often having only a split second in the air to make the right decision about a pass, and being aware that my ability to follow my instincts and control my body came from my core. I would feel it working and stabilizing me, helping me to change my position if I needed to, even in mid-air with the ball in my hand. NBA basketball players today grace the court with their athleticism, acceleration, deceleration, agility and jumping ability, as well as their ball skills and awareness. There is no doubt that the function of these players stems from the core and its associated musculature. It is the capacity of the core that allows the body to complete high-end tasks – changing direction, jumping, shooting, diving, throwing, catching and defending – at such high speeds, and the limbs that complement that core capacity.

The prescription and choice of exercises will depend on many factors, and frequency, sets, reps, duration and load can all be manipulated according to the training experience of the athlete. Are they fit or completing rehabilitation? What are their targets? What phase of training are they in: off-season, pre-season, in-season or competition?

Exercise prescription is not a pure science. The examples above provide some guidance on what may be appropriate, but every athlete is different. The skill of the practitioner or S&C coach lies in completing the needs analysis, selecting the exercises for a reason and with purpose, and establishing an outcome goal. Once this goal has been achieved, it is important for the programme to be developed and progressed to ensure continued adaptation and adherence.

Creativity should be used, too, to produce and design a challenging, smart and fun programme for a client. Considering the requirements of particular sports, and what the client needs to be able to do well, will help the practitioner select exercises to complement any regular strength and conditioning plan and develop a strong, robust athlete who is fit for purpose.

ACUTE AND CHRONIC INJURY: ACUTE TRAUMA AND OVER-USE/OVERLOADING ISSUES AND AGE-SPECIFIC TRAINING

Acute and Chronic Injury

When injury or pain occurs, the first point of contact is often a medical practitioner or doctor. It is important to ensure that the pain is caused by non-specific or mechanical conditions – it may be either gradual or sudden in terms of onset, and it could be the result of lifting something awkwardly, poor posture, or a sprain or strain from sporting activity or an accident, or it may be stress-related. Very rarely, back pain can be a symptom of a more serious problem such as a broken bone in the spine, an infection, cauda equina syndrome (where the nerves in the lower back become severely compressed), or cancer (https://www.nhs.uk/conditions/back-pain/causes).

The medical practitioner or doctor will assess the severity of the condition and provide appropriate advice or medication. Muscle relaxants or pain relief and anti-inflammatories such as ibuprofen may be necessary in acute cases. Ice packs or hot packs may also be recommended, along with exercise classes, such as Pilates, or one-to-one strength and conditioning, or manual therapy, for example with a chiropractor or osteopath, in addition to physiotherapy. The decision of which type of practitioner to use is very personal.

Psychological support and therapies such as cognitive behavioural therapy (CBT) can also help with the management of back pain, by changing how the patient thinks about his or her condition. Pain in the back is of course very real in physical terms, but the way the patient thinks and feels about it can make it worse. For an adult, managing back pain is often a real challenge, becoming not only a physical limitation but also a mental health issue. It can affect work, family life, recreational activities and the individual's general sense of wellbeing and contentment. Having a support network and believing in a solution are essential to aid recovery, as is being confident and brave enough to restart activity and strengthening after pain. Pain is an inhibitor, causing the body to 'shut down', meaning that it does not want to be used. The isometric, early strength and activation exercises are essential for building confidence and trust in anyone who has experienced the debilitating sensation that can result from back pain.

According to Patrick *et al.* (2016), some 80 per cent of the population will at some point experience acute back pain. Treatment of an acute episode of back pain includes relative rest, activity modification, nonsteroidal anti-inflammatories, and physical therapy. Patient education is also vital, as these patients are at risk of further episodes. In their view, chronic back pain (defined as lasting for more than 6 months) develops in a small percentage of patients. They suggest that treatment of these individuals should be supportive, with the goal of reducing pain and improving function (Patrick *et al.*, 2016).

Age-Specific Training

For youth sportspeople and athletes, it is important to coach excellent technique from the start. Good body awareness should be encouraged and bad habits discouraged, with good focus during core and posterior chain training. This age group should be educated on the long-term benefits of such training and not feel like it is a 'filler' in the training day, to keep them at the training ground for longer.

It may be valuable in this youth age group to complete separate foundation exercise sessions specifically to strengthen the core, either as a small group or even as individuals if time allows. Planks, bridging, basic flexion and extension exercises, as well as an introduction to cable, medicine ball or band work, will all be useful. Getting a young person to learn about their body and how it moves is important, as is ensuring that there is a balance between strength development and mobility as this age group grows.

Training load and exposure must also be considered. Often, the best athletes or players are asked to take part in more games or train more frequently than everyone else. It is therefore vital to keep an eye on any individuals who fall into this highly talented category, monitoring their training load and ensuring that rest days are prescribed. The best athletes often end up performing for their school team, their club team, and their county or regional team, as well as for fun with their friends, and overload can be an issue.

Although they may be robust and resilient during adolescence, it is important to ensure good neurological development for young people, and consider long-term athlete development pathways. All components of the pathway must be monitored and managed effectively with the individual in mind, perhaps at the expense of the teams' results. Mobility, strength development (including core strength), nutrition, education, training load, schoolwork, peers, family, friendships and, of course, time off and rest all need to be considered and respected.

As the young athlete grows, it is well worth combining an effective foundation core programme, progressed appropriately once a certain level has been reached, along with a flexibility programme. This should help prevent growth injury, such as Osgood Schlatters or Sever's disease.

Hopefully, the days when a 'core conditioning' session would involve a group of kids doing 50 sit-ups as fast as they could, regardless of technique, are gone, and more attention to detail is given for better outcomes. The case studies show how, by having a strong core, injuries such as groin strains, hamstring tendinopathy and pars defect can be managed, with an improved level of functional strength. This strength development can also be protective and help prevent injury.

In both acute and chronic low back pain episodes, in adults and young people, consideration should be given to the following factors:

- correct diagnosis;
- effective guidance on pain relief;
- appropriate psychological support and awareness of mental wellbeing;
- progressive and appropriate exercise programme and prescription;
- good education to help prevent future problems: posture, correct bad habits, improve body awareness; and
- on-going conditioning.

APPLIED CORE CONDITIONING: PROGRAMMING, PRESCRIPTION

The best way to prevent an onset of low back pain, and avoid other physical problems, is to be fit and conditioned. Everyday tasks – carrying a baby, lifting at work, driving a long-haul vehicle, gardening – as well as sporting activity – lungeing for a tackle in football or hockey or extending to save a goal – all demand correct technique. In addition, good posture, while using the PC, for example, and being aware of how the body moves can all help in prevention. The cost to the economy in terms of lost business hours is significant all over the world; the solution would appear to be a better awareness of back health, movement education and appropriate and improved strength.

CHAPTER 5

SUMMARY

The core is an integrated combination of muscles that can be considered to extend around the midsection of the body, just below the chest, to the midpoint of the thighs. Training it is multi-faceted in nature. Attempting to isolate and encourage activation of the key stabilizer muscles – transverse abdominis, multifidus, external and internal obliques, quadratus lumborum, the erector spinae muscles and glutes, for example – is not particularly functional. In reality, they are difficult to isolate and, in any case, they all work together as a unit.

Once a foundation of strength has been achieved, the programming can become more applied and functional, and any strength gain through the core musculature will become protective. Recent research has shown that Olympic lifts and compound, multi-joint, multi-planar lifts activate the core, posterior chain and lumbo-pelvic musculature. Being very specific, they are a smart choice in relation to exercise selection and will transfer to improved performance, in addition to developing sound core strength.

The time lost by businesses who have employees off work with low back pain represents a significant financial burden. It has been estimated that around 8.9 million working days were lost in Great Britain due to work-related musculoskeletal disorders in 2016–17 (HSE, November 2017). Surely, introducing a wellness package at work, with a foundation core strength programme playing its part in a holistic approach, would result in a healthier group of employees who are fit for purpose.

Education on strength, posture and ergonomics makes a difference to people and outcomes. The Health and Safety Executive has produced a number of online resources to help employers support their staff. There are also a number of private wellness companies who have identified the need to support employees at work, to help with productivity and boost a sense of value at work. Guidance is available on such matters as manual handling, risk assessment in pushing and pulling, and making the best use of manual handling aids. There are also regulations on display screen equipment, which has been shown to increase the risk of musculoskeletal disorders, visual fatigue and mental stress. It is positive that these vulnerable areas are being identified in the workplace, and some employers are addressing this as the population ages and illness and injury are more prevalent.

I do believe that every individual has a responsibility to be fit for purpose as well. The facts are that the risk of low back pain increases with ageing, and 80 per cent of the population will suffer an episode of low back pain, so surely a prophylactic approach is wise. The benefits of a solid applied core programme are evident. The case studies all demonstrate a positive outcome and some of these clients had been in chronic pain for a number of years. Becoming stronger really helped their outcome.

SUMMARY

Becoming stronger through the core creates a more robust kinetic chain and the result is a reduction in injury potential. Whole-body movements that demand strength and stability through the core will enhance the body's capacity for load and allow for the positive management of the physical demands placed upon it, thereby helping to reduce the incidence of injury. A conditioned body is a more capable one.

I always tell my injured clients that they will finish my conditioning programme a better, stronger, more educated individual than they were when they first arrived. Sometimes, an injury can be a blessing in disguise, if an individual becomes stronger and more resilient and robust because of an effective strengthening programme. The long-term gain can be worth the blip at the beginning.

My mum is in her mid-70s and has just started a weekly Pilates class. She really enjoys it, has an hour of 'me' time and already feels stronger through her core, low back and glutes 6 weeks into the programme. This will help her long-term strength and functional capacity as she ages. She is very active with her grandchildren, she plays golf, goes bowling and rides a stationary bike daily, amongst other things. It is fantastic that she has taken the initiative and is responsible for her own health. She wants to be active and strong and able. Many people take it for granted that they will have a healthy, fit body as they age. It is a wonderful thing, but it is something to be respected and everyone should be more proactive in order to be protective.

There is also no doubt that physical activity helps with metal health and wellbeing, as it increases the release of endorphins. The link between pain and depression has become clearly established as awareness of mental health issues has increased. Creating a healthier nation and reducing the incidence of low back pain can help address those issues. In reviewing the benefits of exercise, Sharma *et al.* (2006) summarized that exercise improves mental health by reducing anxiety, depression and negative mood, and by improving cognitive function. Exercise has also been found to alleviate symptoms such as low self-esteem and social withdrawal (Sharma *et al.*, 2006).

Maybe prescribing two to three exercises, to be completed a few times a week, to the general population, as I did for the 40-year-old MRI scan client who had severe low back pain, would result in a decrease in the risk of low back pain and an improvement in mental health. It would also reduce this burden on the workplace, the health system, the individual's family, and on the individuals themselves.

As far as athletes are concerned, core conditioning has been a part of their conditioning programme structure for many years. Having worked with many different athletes and teams, I have come to the conclusion that there is a definite link between strengthening the core, the posterior chain and the sling systems and a positive physical outcome, injury

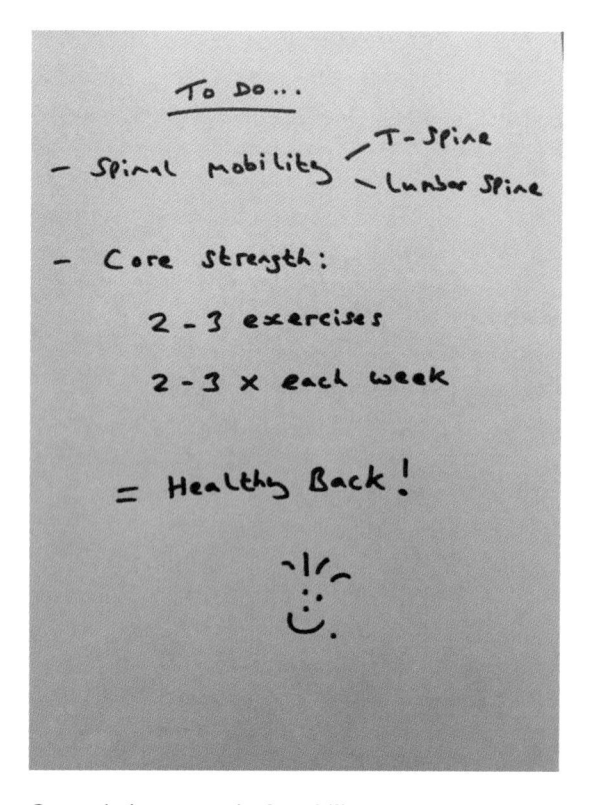

Committing to a spinal mobility and core strengthening programme on a regular basis will undoubtedly pay dividends in the prevention of low back pain.

SUMMARY

prevention and performance benefits. A stronger core takes the load off the hamstrings, quads, calves, hip flexors and groins, all of which may be more susceptible to muscular injury. I had one client who had plantar fasciitis who, after review, was identified as having a weak posterior chain. As his posterior chain was made stronger through core, lumbo-pelvic and loaded posterior chain work, including dead lift, Romanian dead lift, supine Swiss ball bridging, and so on, his foot pain went away. The body really is a kinetic chain, all linked together.

The development and delivery of applied conditioning for a strong and stable core musculature for everyone should be designed as follows:

1. Foundation exercises.
2. Functional and sports-specific exercise selection and progressions.
3. Mastery: super-set sports-specific exercise with drills, increased intensity and loading, recognizing the value of Olympic lifts and compound exercises.

Programming for the high-performance athlete will probably rotate between the top, middle and bottom of the pyramid, depending on the training phase and the need to vary the training stimulus, but always with a physiological overload. However, the foundation level – the base of the pyramid – is required for everyone, from the construction worker to the recreational weekend sports person, from the professional athlete to my 70-year-old mum! There is no point cutting corners here: control, body awareness and subsequent overload from the stimulus and appropriate progression are all required. Strength is protective.

By applying a few core exercises into a daily routine, or progressing all the way to a comprehensive, thorough applied strength and conditioning programme, every individual can make a conscious choice to become better equipped for daily living and sports performance. Following injury or illness, there may be a need to start over again with the foundation level, but it is important to believe that it is possible to return to pre-injury levels, or even

Mastery:
super set sport specific exercise with specific sports drills: Increased Intensity and Loading

Functional & Sport Specific Exercise Selection

Foundation Exercises: Isometric, Activation, Body Awareness, Breathing, Bracing and Control

exceed them. It will take a bit of work, but the results will happen and will be beneficial.

My hope is that this book will inspire effective programming and prescription, and motivate everyone to be fit for purpose, with the appreciation that core strength has a vital role to play in the prevention of injury as well as in effective performance. Ironically, my back is sore from sitting and writing this book. I think I need to go and do some spinal mobility and strengthening work...!

GLOSSARY

Agonist and antagonist muscles: an agonist muscle is a contracting muscle whose contraction is opposed by another muscle (an antagonist). The antagonist muscle counteracts the action of the agonist. For example, biceps and triceps work together as agonists and antagonist muscles.

Appendicular skeleton: the bones that make up the shoulder girdle, upper extremities, pelvis, and lower extremities.

Axial skeleton: the bones of the head and trunk.

Cerebrospinal fluid: the clear watery fluid that fills the space between the arachnoid membrane and the pia mater.

Concentric muscle action: muscle contraction resulting in its shortening.

Delayed onset muscle soreness (DOMS): the muscular pain and soreness felt several hours to days after unaccustomed or strenuous exercise. The soreness is typically more intense around 24 to 72 hours after exercise.

Eccentric muscle action: elongation of a muscle where it acts to decelerate the joint at the end of a movement or control the repositioning of a load.

Fascia: a sheet of connective tissue surrounding muscles, bones, organs, nerves, blood vessels and other structures within the body.

Grade I muscle strain: the result of an overstretching of the muscle or tendon. Small tears to muscle fibres may or may not occur. There may be mild pain, with or without swelling.

Grade II muscle strain: an overstretching of the muscle or its tendon, with more of the fibres torn but not completely ruptured. Symptoms may include pain with swelling. The injury site is tender. Bruising may occur if small blood vessels at the site of injury are damaged as well. Movement may be difficult because of pain and swelling.

Grade III muscle strain: in many cases, many or indeed all of the muscle fibres are torn or ruptured. Pain, swelling, tenderness and bruising are usually present. Movement is usually very difficult.

Isometric muscle action: muscle contraction without a shortening or change in length between its origin and insertion.

Kinetic chain: term used to describe how forces occur during human motion and how segments of the body are linked together.

Meninges: the three membranes (the dura mater, arachnoid, and pia mater) that line the skull and vertebral canal and enclose the brain and spinal cord.

Pilates: an exercise regime typically performed with the use of specialized apparatus and designed to improve the overall condition of the body.

Proprioceptors: sensory receptors in muscles, joint capsules and surrounding tissues that signal information to the central nervous system about the position and movement of body parts. An example would be the angle at a joint or the length of a muscle.

Range of movement (ROM): the measurement of movement around a specific joint or body part.

Smooth muscle: an involuntary non-striated muscle, found within the walls of blood vessels, lymphatic vessels, the urinary bladder, uterus, male and female reproductive tracts and the gastrointestinal tract.

Spinal cord: the cylindrical bundle of nerve fibres and associated tissue that is enclosed in the spine and connects nearly all parts of the body to the brain, with which it forms the central nervous system.

Stretch-Shortening Cycle (SSC): the 'pre-stretch' action that is commonly observed during typical human movements such as jumping and bounding. An eccentric muscle contraction followed immediately by a concentric contraction of the same muscle group is an example of this pre-stretch, which allows the athlete to produce more force and move quicker. It can be trained with plyometric (jumping-based) activities.

Vertebrae: bones that support the body and provide the protective bony corridor through which the spinal cord passes. The 26 bones that make up the spine differ considerably in size and structure according to location. There are 7 cervical vertebrae, 12 thoracic, 5 lumbar, 1 sacral and 1 coccyx.

REFERENCES

Arokoski JP, Valta T, Airaksinen O, Kankaanpaa M. Back and abdominal muscle function during stabilization exercises. *Arch Phys Med Rehabilitation* 82: 1089–1098, 2001.

Ashish Sharma, MD, Vishal Madaan, MD and Frederick, D, Petty, MD, Ph.D. Exercise for Mental Health. *The Primary Care Companion Journal of Clinical Psychiatry*. 2006; 8(2): 106.

Axial and appendicular skeleton: http://medicaldictionary.thefreedictionary.com/axial+skeleton

Fascia Research Congress (2009) *Terminology Used in Fascia Research*. Available from: http://www.fasciacongress.org/2009/glossary.htm [Accessed 5 April 2012]

Babalola JF, Awolola OE, Hamzat TK. *African Journal for Physical Health Education, Recreation and Dance*, Volume 14, Issue 2, Jun 2008, pp. 188–198.

Borg G. (1998) Borg's perceived exertion and pain scales. *Human Kinetics*.

BrianMac Sports Coach: http://www.brianmac.co.uk

Causes of back pain: https://www.nhs.uk/conditions/back-pain/causes

Delayed Onset Muscle Soreness (DOMS): Reprinted with permission of the American College of Sports Medicine. Copyright © 2011 American College of Sports Medicine.

Denniger JW, Mahal Y, and Merens W et al. The relationship between somatic symptoms and depression. New Research Abstracts of the 155th annual meeting of the American Psychiatric Association. 21 May 2002 Philadelphia, Pa. Abstract NR251:68–69.

Diastasis recti, or divarication: https://www.nhs.uk/Conditions/pregnancy-and-baby/Pages/yourbody-after-childbirth.aspx

'ergonomic'. *Collins English Dictionary – Complete and Unabridged 10th Edition*. HarperCollins Publishers. 7 Nov. 2017. (dictionary.com. browse/ergonomic)

Fisher K, Johnston M. (1997) Validation of the ODQ, its sensitivity as a measure of change following treatment and its relationship with other aspects of the chronic pain experience. *Physiotherapy Theory and Practice* 13, 67–80

Fredericson M, Moore T. Core stabilisation training for middle and long-distance runners. *Physical Medicine and Rehabilitation Clinics of North America*, volume 16, issue 3. August 2005, pages 669–689.

Gottschall JS, Mills J, and Hastings B. Integration Core Exercises Elicit Greater Muscle Activation than Isolation Exercises. *Journal of Strength and Conditioning Research*, 27(3), 590–596. March 2013.

Grenier SG, McGill SM. Quantification of Lumbar Stability by Using 2 Different Abdominal Activation Strategies. *Arch Phys Med Rehabilitation* Vol 88, January 2007.

Groin strain: http://www.sportsinjuryclinic.net/sport-injuries/hip-groin-pain/groin-strain

REFERENCES

Hawkins RD, Hulse MA, Wilkinson C, Hodson A, Gibson M. The association football medical research programme: an audit of injuries in professional football. *Br J Sports Med.* 2001 Feb;35(1):43-7.

Health and Safety at Work Summary statistics for Great Britain 2017 © Crown copyright 2017. Health and Safety Executive. November 2017.

Henschke N, Maher CG, Refshauge KM, et al. Prevalence of and screening for serious spinal pathology in patients presenting to primary care settings with acute low back pain. *Arthritis Rheum* 2009;60:3072–80.

Herniated or slipped disc: https://www.nhs.uk/conditions/slipped-disc

Hodges PW, Richardson CA. Altered trunk muscle recruitment in people with low back pain with upper limb movement at different speeds. *Arch Phys Med Rehabilitation* 1999;80:1005-12.

Injury grading (grade I, grade II or grade III): www.physioroom.com

John Rusin, DPT, PT, CSCS, Scotty Butcher. Core Strength and Functionality with Loaded Carries. NSCA COACH 4.3, NSCA.COM.

Juan Carlos Santana, MEd, CSCS. National Strength and Conditioning Association, *Journal of Strength and Conditioning* Volume 25, Number 2, pages 73–74, 2003.

Kavcic N, Grenier S, McGill SM. Determining the stabilizing role of individual torso muscles during rehabilitation exercises. *Spine* (Phila Pa 1976). 2004 Jun 1;29(11):1254-65.

Khan KM, Cook JL, Bonar F, Harcourt P, Astrom M. (1999) Histopathology of common tendinopathies. *Sports Med* 27: 393–408.

Kinetic chain: https://medical-dictionary.thefreedictionary.com/kinetic+chain+exercise

Koes BW, van Tulder M, Lin C-WC, Macedo LG, McAuley J, Maher C. An updated overview of clinical guidelines for the management of non-specific low back pain in primary care. *Eur Spine J* 2010;19:2075–94.

Koes BW, van Tulder MW, Thomas S. Diagnosis and treatment of low back pain. *BMJ* 2006;332: 1430–34.

Kopec JA, Esdaile JM, Abrahamowicz M, Abenhaim L, Wood-Dauphinee S, Lamping DL, Williams JI. The Quebec Back Pain Disability Scale. Measurement properties. *Spine* (Phila Pa 1976). 1995 Feb 1;20(3):341–52.

Labour Force Survey and RIDDOR for 2014–15 and 2016–17, and HSE Costs to Britain Model. © Crown copyright 2017. Published by the Health and Safety Executive November 2017. *Contains public sector information licensed under the Open Government Licence v3.0.*

Madhukar H, Trivedi MD. The Link Between Depression and Physical Symptoms. *Primary Care Companion Journal of Clinical Psychiatry.* 2004; 6 (suppl 1): 12–16.

McGill S. Core training: Evidence translating to better performance and injury prevention. *Strength Conditioning Journal*, 32: 33–46, 2010.

Moseley GL, Hodges PW, Gandevia SC. Deep and superficial fibers of the lumbar multifidus muscle are differentially active during voluntary arm movements. *Spine* (Phila Pa 1976). 2002 Jan 15;27(2): E29-36.

The National Institute of Neurological Disorders and Stroke. Back Pain Fact Sheet, NINDS, December 2014. NIH Publication No. 15-5161. https://www.ninds.nih.gov/Disorders/Patient-Caregiver-Education/Fact-Sheets/Low-Back-Pain-Fact-Sheet

The National Strength and Conditioning Association. Essentials of Strength Training and Conditioning, *Human Kinetics*; 2 edition (July 27, 2000).

Nicole Nelson, MS, LMT. Diaphragmatic Breathing: The Foundation of Core Stability. *National Strength and Conditioning Association.* Volume 34(5), October 2012.

Nuzzo JL, McCaulley GO, Cormie P, Cavill MJ, and McBride JM. Trunk Muscle Activity During Stability Ball and Free Weight Exercises. *Journal of Strength and Conditioning Research*, 22(1), 95–102. January 2008.

REFERENCES

Pars defect/spondylolisthesis: https://www.nhs.uk/conditions/spondylolisthesis

Patrick N, Emanski E, Knaub MA. Acute and Chronic Low Back Pain. *The Medical Clinics of North America*. 2016 Jan;100(1):169-81. doi: 10.10.16/j.mcna.2015.08.015.

Pelvic floor: American Society of colon and rectal surgeons: https://www.fascrs.org/patients/diseasecondition/pelvic-floor-dysfunction-expanded-version

Pelvic floor exercises: https://www.nhs.uk

Piriformis syndrome: http://www.gloshospitals.nhs.uk/en/Wards-and-Departments/Departments/Pain-Management/Different-Pains/Nerve-Pain/Types-of-Nerve-Pain/Nerve-Entrapment/Piriformis-Syndrome/

Richardson CA, Snijders CJ, Hides JA, Damen L, Pas MS, and Storm J. The relation between the transversus abdominis muscles, sacroiliac joint mechanics, and low back pain. *Spine*. 2002; 27: 399–405

Roland, MO, Morris, RW. A study of the natural history of back pain. Chapter 1: Development of a reliable and sensitive measure of disability in low back pain. *Spine* 1983; 8: 141–144.

Serape effect: https://en.wikipedia.org/wiki/Serape_effect

Shadab Uddin, Fuzail Ahmed. Effect of Lumbar Stabilization exercises versus pressure feedback training in low back ache patients, *European Scientific Journal*, Jul 2013. 1st Annual International Interdisciplinary Conference, AIIC 2013, 24–26 April, Azores, Portugal.

Silfies SP, Mehta R, Smith SS, Karduna AR. Differences in feedforward trunk muscle activity in subgroups of patients with mechanical low back pain. *Arch Phys Med Rehabilitation* 2009;90:1159-69.

Spinal cord: http://www.bbc.co.uk/science/humanbody/body/factfiles/spinalcord/spinal_cord.shtml

STarT Back Screening Tool: https://www.keele.ac.uk/sbst/startbacktool

Vern Gambetta, Athletic Development Defining the Discipline, The Gain Network, 2007.

Wilson Dr Fiona, Back pain in rowing – update on current understanding, 02 MAY 2016 World Rowing: http://www.worldrowing.com/news/back-pain-rowing-update-current-understanding

INDEX

activating the core 29
acute and chronic injury 162
age-specific training 163
adductor/groin strain case study 96
alternating hip flexion extension 53, 154
appendicular skeleton 11
assessment 36, 38
axial skeleton 11

band diagonal lunge walk 80
band hip abduction 51, 80
band hip extension 61
band hip flexion 61
band rotation 128
band walks 69, 148
barbell 116, 127
biceps curl 13
bilateral hamstring tendinopathy case study 75
body blade rotation 147
BOSU alternating hip flexion-extension 157
BOSU medicine ball rotation 62, 150
BOSU medicine ball throw 130
BOSU supine isometric stabilization 72
box bridging with isometric ball holds 92
bracing 30
breathing 30

cable hip abduction/adduction 106
cable hip flexion/extension 106
cable rotation 115, 128, 130, 132

cable shuffle 142
cable straight-arm lateral pull-down 157
calf self-massage 79
cardiac muscle 12, 14
cervical region 21
chest press rotation 116
clam 50, 93
close the gate 98
closed chain exercises 24
concentric exercise 16
concentric loading 114
conditioning 123
coordination 32
core musculature 26
crawler 60

dead lift 143, 149
deep lateral rotator muscles 19
diagonal walker 57
double-leg bridging 90, 102, 112
dumbbell lateral pullover 84

eccentric exercise 16
eccentric loading 114
endurance-based exercise 118
endurance events 152
erector spinae muscles 20

fascia 14
fibre types 15

INDEX

financial cost 34
focus pads 131
force-velocity curve 122
forward prone walk 114
four-point stabilization 92

glute band activation 57, 68, 80
glute self-massage 67, 79
glute-ham raise 84, 140
good morning exercise 85
grades of muscular injury 96
groin mobility 98

hamstring heel flicks 85
hamstring self-massage 78
hang clean pull 139
high pull 158
hip 17
hip external rotation stretch 101
hip flexion abduction 91, 99
hip flexion cable extension 142
hip flexion cable rotation 62
hip flexion rotation 156
hip internal rotation stretch 101
hip mobility 98
hip rotation 73

iliopsoas muscles 18
innervation 20
internal and external rotation 99
isometric exercise 16, 118
isometric strength 112
ITB self-massage 68, 79

Keele STarT Back Screening Tool 37
kettle bell swing 139
key muscles of the trunk and spine 17
kinetic chain 24
kneeling arm-leg raise 53, 59, 91
kneeling cable push press 94
kneeling cable rotation 95
Kraus Weber Test 39

lateral bound rotation 129
lateral jump acceleration 141
lateral lunch step-down with wood-chop rotation 104
lateral lunge hip flexion 100
lateral step-up with hip flexion 104
left and right sidewalks 57
linear events 152
loaded sit-up 17
loads in training 30
long lever 51
lumbar region 21
lumbar spine 22
lunge walk rotation 135, 158

medicine ball 17, 105, 116, 120, 126, 135, 136, 148, 149, 150
MRI scan 22
multi-directional high-intensity intermittent sports 132
multi-directional lunges 107
muscular imbalance 36
muscular system 10
muscular testing 34
musculature of the sling system 27

needs analysis 44
nervous system 21
NSCA resistance training guidelines 122

open chain exercises 24
open the gate 99
Oswestry Low Back Pain Disability Questionnaire 37
over-use/overloading issues 162

paddle 147
pars defect: spondylolisthesis case study 55
patient questionnaire 37
pelvic floor exercises 89
pelvic girdle 17
periformis syndrome case study 64
plank 17, 51
plank arm-raise 83

INDEX

plank hold 118
posterior chain 28
post-partum diastasis recti case study 87
power-based exercise 120
prescription 112, 116
programme design 123, 161
programming 112
prolapsed/herniated disc case study 48
prone hip extension 59, 72
prone kneeling hip extension 114
prone walk 151

quad self-massage 78
Quebec Back Pain Disability Scale 37

rating of perceived exertion 45
risk 34
Roland-Morris Disability Questionnaire 37
Roman chair back extension 138
rotation sports 124

sacral region 21
seated cable crunch rotation 131, 150
seated events 144
seated spinal rotation 129
seated wood chop 148
serape effect 28
side laying stabilization 113
side-lying hip extension 100
single leg Swiss ball curls 115
single-leg bridging 52, 58, 68, 81, 113, 103, 156
single-leg cable rotation 130
single-leg front step-up 81

single-leg lateral step-up 82
single-leg split good morning exercise 71
single-leg straight-leg dead lift 140
single-leg triceps extension push-up 155
skeletal muscle 12, 14
skeletal system 10
sling system 25, 27
slump test 38
smooth muscle 14
spinal column 18, 20
split clean 141
split jump rotation 126, 129, 131, 135, 157
split squat 103
sports-specific training and prescription 116
sports-specific conditioning and programme design 123
stability 32
stability ball 159
stability disc 159
stabilization rotation 125
standing spinal self-massage 68
step-down stabilization 83
straight-leg Romanian dead lift 70, 82, 105
supine stabilization 113
Swiss ball 52, 58, 70, 94, 103, 127, 136, 137, 146, 154, 155, 156, 158

thoracic regions 21
trunk 18
trunk muscle coordination 28
tyre rotation 131

wood chop 126